AT LAST—THE RIGHT CUTS AT THE RIGHT PRICE!

Haircutting was never simpler! With this fully illustrated guide to fashionable at-home hairstyling, *anyone*, no matter how inexperienced, can cut hair with the precision of a professional stylist.

Cutting Hair at Home puts all the right tools in your hands and a world of styling options at your fingertips. Whether you choose a sophisticated bob or a layered look, whether you're cutting a new-wave style or a child's quick clip, these mistake-proof instructions ensure that your every cut will come out as you intended. Great looks don't have to be expensive. Now you can cut *anybody's* hair—family, friends, even your own—while trimming your hair-care costs to practically zero!

CUTTING HAIR AT HOME

LEE POLA, a professional hairstylist, has her own salon in New York City. PATRICIA BOZIC is the author of several hair and fashion books.

CUTTING HAIR AT HOME

STEP-BY-STEP HAIRCUTTING FOR EVERYONE

Patricia Bozic and Lee Pola

Illustrations by Jack Eckstein

Produced by The Miller Press, Inc.

A PLUME BOOK

NEW AMERICAN LIBRARY

NEW YORK AND SCARBOROUGH, ONTARIO

PLUME TRADEMARK REG. U.S. PAT. OFF. AND FOREIGN COUNTRIES
REG. TRADEMARK—MARCA REGISTRADA
HECHO EN WESTFORD, MASS., U.S.A.

SIGNET, SIGNET CLASSIC, MENTOR, PLUME, MERIDIAN and NAL BOOKS
are published *in the United States* by New American Library
1633 Broadway, New York, New York 10019,
in Canada by the New American Library of Canada Limited,
81 Mack Avenue, Scarborough, Ontario M1L 1M8

Library of Congress Cataloging-in-Publication Data

Pola, Lee.
Cutting hair at home.

1. Haircutting. I. Bozic, Patricia.
II. Title.
TT970.P65   1986   646.7′242   86-8348
ISBN 0-452-25830-8 (pbk.)
First Printing, July, 1986

1 2 3 4 5 6 7 8 9

PRINTED IN THE UNITED STATES OF AMERICA

CONTENTS

**INTRODUCTION: CUT YOUR
HAIR LIKE A PRO**   15

1 **THE BASICS**   17
CLEANSING   17
    Hair Massage   18
    Shampooing   18
    Dandruff   19
CONDITIONING   19
THE HAIR CARE REGIMEN THAT'S RIGHT
    FOR YOU   20
BRUSHING   22
HAIR HELPERS   23
    Tools   23
    Mousses and Gels   24
CLASSIC BLOW-DRYING TECHNIQUE   25
    Quickie Blow-Dry   26
    Blow-Drying Tips   26

2 **SETTING UP SHOP**   29
ASSEMBLE YOUR TOOLS   29
FIFTEEN PRO TIPS   32
SPECIAL HAIRCUTTING PROBLEMS—
    LICKING THAT COWLICK   35
PRECUT PROCEDURES   37

3 PRECISION HAIRCUTTING 39

HAIRCUTTING AND STYLING FOR WOMEN 40
  Choosing a Flattering Style 40
    Go With Your Hair Type and Texture 40
    Analyze Your Face Shape 41
    The Perfect Proportion 43
  Blunt Cuts 43
    Long Hair 43
    Foolproof Way to Cut Bangs 48
    The Bob 52
  Layered Cuts 56
    Long Hair 56
    Short Hair 63
    The Modern Cut for Wavy to Curly Hair 69
    Growing Out Your Hair—How to Go from
      Layered to All One Length 75
HAIRCUTTING AND STYLING FOR MEN 80
  Men's Layered Cut 80
  Modified Military Cut 85
  Fringe Benefits—How to Care for a Mustache
    and Beard 88
    Mustaches 89
    Beards 89
  How to Hide or Disguise That Bald or
  Thin Spot 91
HAIRCUTTING AND STYLING FOR CHILDREN
AND TEENS 92
  Taking Care of Baby 92
  No-Fuss Cuts for Toddlers 93
    Tips on Taming a Toddler During a Haircut 93
    The Quick One-Step Cut 93
    The Bowl Cut 97
    Hair Repair Cut 101
  Hair Care for Teens 104
    For Girls Only—Styling Tips 105

4 SPECIAL EFFECTS — 111

PERFECT PERMS — 111
  Perm Checklist — 112
  Home Perm Tips — 112
  Maintaining a Perm — 114
  Perm Problems — 114
  Perming Color-Treated Hair — 114
RELAXING HAIR — 115
HAIR COLORING CUES — 116
  Temporary Rinses — 117
  Semipermanent and Permanent Hair Colors — 117
  Choosing the Right Shade — 118
  Highlighting and Hair Painting — 118
  Frosting — 118
  Get Your Hair Glowing — 119
  Hair Lighteners — 119
  Henna — 119
    Henna How–Tos — 120
  Care for Color-Treated Hair — 121

QUESTIONS AND ANSWERS — 123

Acknowledgments

Special thanks to our consultants: Julian Garcia of Glemby's at B. Altman & Co., New York, for information on black hair care; and Lynnette Schaller of Le Salon, New York, for background information on hair color and perms. We'd also like to express our gratitude to our models: Karen, Steven, Laurie, Robin and Susan.

CUTTING HAIR
AT HOME

Introduction: Cut Your Hair Like a Pro

Even if you have no experience cutting hair, you can master the basic techniques in this book. The instructions and accompanying diagrams were developed with a professional hairstylist, and will guide you through each haircut step by step. We've included great cuts that are flattering and up-to-date and fall into place with no fuss. There is a style to suit every taste and hair texture—from straight and fine to thick and curly—from old favorites like the blunt cut to sophisticated layered cuts for long and short hair. If you want to start out the easy way and just cut bangs, you'll find directions for a full, thick fringe and the wispy, layered kind. For men, there's a basic, layered cut and a modern military style, plus tips on trimming a mustache and beard. Kids will look neat and cute in the two classic cuts we've included. You'll also find directions for fixing a common hair disaster: when a tot takes scissors to hair and chops off a large piece.

There's something for everyone in this book. We've spelled out the basics for you: how to choose the right shampoo and conditioner and the styling aids to use. We've included all you'll need to know about special situations such as washing an infant's hair. There are tips for teens on how to control excessively oily hair. If you want to get rid of gray or brighten blond hair, we've got the how-tos. Our camouflage tricks can help men's thinning hair look thicker. And this book is loaded with quick, easy ways to give your hair a new twist for day or night.

You'll discover that haircutting isn't hard once you get the hang of it. Some cuts are so simple you can do them alone. For others, you'll need a partner to help you. Or you can always have your hairdresser cut your hair according to our instructions. Mastering all the haircuts in this book is worth the effort. You will be well coiffed and you'll have more money in the bank at the end of the year. And that's no small accomplishment.

THE BASICS

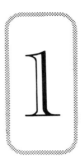

$\mathbf{A}$ clean, shiny head of hair is the best way to flaunt a fabulous haircut. But don't expect a haircut to cure hair that's in poor condition. Good hair care is a must for appearance's sake, but more importantly, it's a factor in maintaining good health. The scalp is, after all, skin and deserves the same amount of attention as your face.

Shampooing your hair and running a comb through it afterward won't be enough to keep it in top form. A consistent program of care is necessary because everyday wear and tear takes a toll on the hair. The things you do to it every day—such as blow-drying, brushing, and using hot rollers—can, over time, damage the hair, resulting in split ends and dryness. Overexposure to the sun can also deprive the hair of oils, leaving it dull and brittle. Hair that's been processed with color or permed also needs extra protection.

Following are the basics that everyone should know about hair care—from choosing the right shampoo and conditioner to the tools that the pros use for styling hair. Children's hair requires special care and will be covered with greater detail in Chapter 3.

Cleansing

You should wash your hair daily with a mild, pH-balanced shampoo formulated for your hair type—normal, oily or dry (see the chart on pages 20-21 for the shampoo that's right for you). Harsh detergent-based shampoos can strip the hair of its natural oils and make it look dull. Even the best shampoo, however, won't get your hair clean if you don't use it properly. Here's how to get your hair whistle clean.

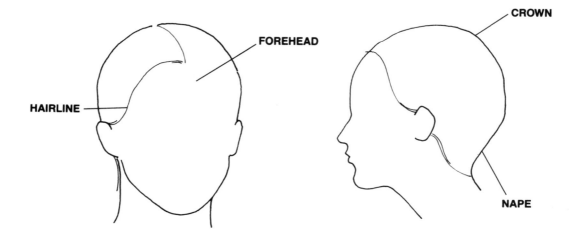

HAIR MASSAGE

Before shampooing, massage the scalp. It only takes a few minutes to do. Massage loosens dirt and oils so they can be washed out of the hair and keeps the scalp in good condition.

Starting anywhere, press your scalp with your fingertips and massage it with a light circular motion. Cover every inch of the scalp, making sure to massage all around the hairline at the front, sides and nape of the neck. Then brush the hair to remove dirt.

SHAMPOOING

1. Wet the hair thoroughly and apply a dab of shampoo.
2. Using the pads of your fingertips, work the shampoo into your scalp, all around the hairline and then out to the ends of the hair. One sudsing is usually enough unless your hair is very dirty. Don't dig into the scalp with your fingernails when washing your hair—you could scratch it. Also avoid rubbing vigorously, which can break the hair.
3. Rinse your hair well. Rinsing should take just as long as shampooing. When you think you've rinsed your hair enough, rinse again to get out every trace of shampoo. Residue from suds can leave a dull film on the hair.

DANDRUFF

If you have it, you'll know it. The main symptoms of dandruff are oiliness, itching and flaking of the scalp. A more serious type of dandruff, called seborrheic dermatitis, is accompanied by redness and inflammation of the scalp and skin. Dandruff isn't contagious, so you can't get it by using someone else's comb or brush.

No one is sure exactly what causes dandruff. What is known is that dandruff occurs when the skin cells on the scalp are shed faster than normal. The cells clump together, forming white flakes, and cling to the scalp or fall onto the shoulders. Stress can also cause a flare-up of dandruff. To get rid of dandruff, you should use a tar-based shampoo. See the chart on pages 20-21 for how to apply it. If the condition doesn't clear up or if you think you have a severe case, you should see a dermatologist.

Conditioning

Conditioning protects your hair from damage, makes it easier to manage and brings out its natural sheen. It's especially important for medium to long hair. Short hair, because it's cut so frequently, doesn't need as much conditioning. For hair to shine, the cuticle (the outer covering of the hair shaft, made up of tiny cells resembling shingles on a roof) must lie flat. Light bounces off this smooth surface and makes hair look lustrous. But when the cuticle is frayed, it won't reflect as much light and will appear drab.

Conditioners aren't for women only. Men with dry, fine, frizzy or thinning hair will have more control over their hair if they use conditioners regularly.

There are two types of conditioners—instant and deep-penetrating. You should use an instant conditioner after every shampoo. An instant conditioner removes snarls and gives the hair a smooth, shiny appearance. Most instant conditioners are left on the hair for one minute. If your hair needs more conditioning, you can get a richer instant conditioner that you leave on for five minutes.

A deep conditioner is the remedy for hair that's dry or damaged. And when used regularly, it will keep hair at its healthiest. The active ingredient in a deep conditioner is protein, which permeates the hair shaft and strengthens it. It also adds mois-

Hair Type, Texture or Condition	Characteristics	Shampoo	Conditioner
NORMAL	Your hair stays fresh between shampoos and doesn't droop or look oily.	A formula for normal hair.	Light instant conditioner or finishing rinse after every shampoo. Deep conditioner once a month.
DRY	Hair can look dull, snarls easily and may be split on the ends.	An extra-mild moisturizing shampoo for dry hair.	A rich instant conditioner after every shampoo. A deep conditioner every two weeks.
OILY	Hair looks limp and greasy between washings.	A shampoo for oily hair or an oil-free formula. Wash your hair twice daily if necessary to control oiliness.	An oil-free cream or finishing rinse or a lightweight oil-free conditioner. If hair ends are dry, use a deep conditioner on them, but keep it off your scalp.
FINE HAIR	Feels silky to the touch. Looks limp and lacks body. It may be a mass of tangles after shampooing. Fine curly hair tends to be frizzy.	A body-building shampoo with protein or a formula for "extra body."	A lightweight instant conditioner that boosts body or that provides "extra body."

Hair Type, Texture or Condition	Characteristics	Shampoo	Conditioner
COARSE HAIR	Your hair is wiry and hard to get a comb through. It might become harder to control during humid weather.	Coarse hair tends to be dry. Use a moisturizing shampoo.	A rich instant conditioner. Deep conditioner every two weeks to a month, depending upon how dry your hair is.
DAMAGED	Your hair is very dry and may be split, brittle or broken. It doesn't shine.	A moisturizing shampoo for dry hair. Do not wash your hair more than once a day.	A rich instant conditioner after every shampoo and a deep conditioner once a week. If your hair is badly damaged, use a deep conditioner after every shampoo until the problem improves.
DANDRUFF	The scalp is oily and flaky.	Apply a tar-based shampoo to the scalp only. Gently work it into the scalp to remove scales and leave on for the amount of time specified on the package. Then rinse it out and wash the hair with a mild shampoo. Do daily until the condition improves.	Use a finishing rinse to detangle hair if necessary.

ture to the hair to restore resilience and shine. Deep conditioners are creamy in texture. Comb the conditioner in from the roots to the ends of the hair and leave it on for 10 to 30 minutes. For more penetrating action, you can wrap your hair in a plastic bag. You should deep-condition your hair about once a month to keep it lustrous, especially if you have long hair which is prone to split ends. Oily hair is the exception to this rule—it has enough oil of its own and doesn't usually need deep conditioning, except perhaps on the ends. If your hair is badly damaged, you might want to deep-condition it more than once a month to bring it back to health.

Cream or finishing rinses are used to make the hair more manageable. They're great for unsnarling fine hair or children's hair after shampooing. Some contain conditioners, but most do not. The package label will tell you whether or not the rinse has built-in conditioning action.

It's important to use a conditioner or rinse that's suited to your hair type. A conditioner that's too rich for your hair can leave it looking lank and greasy.

Brushing

Daily brushing should be part of your basic hair care program, too. When you brush, oils from the roots of the hair reach the ends. Brushing also revs up circulation in the scalp. Brush your hair for a few minutes each day. Overbrushing can do more damage than good and will split or break your hair. A large, flat brush about 3 inches in diameter with plastic bristles and a foam-rubber base is kindest to the hair.

The correct way to brush the hair is from the bottom up. With your head bent forward, brush from the center of the nape to the hairline in the front of the head and all the way out to the ends. Then brush the sections of hair on each side of the nape the same way. The brush should lightly graze the scalp, not scrape it. Also avoid brushing the hair when it's wet. Wet hair is stretched to its maximum elasticity, and hard brushing can break it.

Hair Helpers

TOOLS

You don't need an arsenal of equipment to style your hair the way it's done at the salon, but a few tools can help you keep your hair in good shape. The items you'll need depend upon what type of hair you have and how you wear it. Here are some recommendations.

Blow-dryer Blow-drying can help you achieve a smooth, sleek look and add volume to the hair. A 1200-watt dryer with two or more settings is best. Look for a lightweight model that's easy to handle.

Diffuser For wavy, curly or permed hair, you can buy an attachment called a diffuser that fits onto the nozzle of a blow-dryer. It sends out a gentle stream of air that won't flatten out waves or curls.

Styling Brushes A round, plastic-bristled brush with a foam-rubber base is best to use with a blow-dryer. It's lightweight and flexible, and the plastic bristles are built to withstand the heat. Styling brushes range in size from 1 to 2½ inches in diameter. The larger the brush, the straighter your hair will turn out.

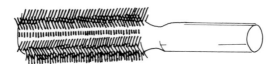

A large round brush about 2 to 2½ inches in diameter is for drying straight hair.

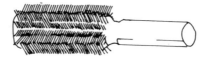

A medium-sized brush, 1½ inches in circumference, will help you create soft waves or curls.

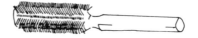

A small circular brush about 1 inch in diameter is for styling tight, springy curls.

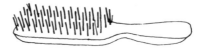

A vent brush has widely spaced teeth that fluff up the hair and give it maximum volume. It's especially good if you have thick wavy, curly or permed hair.

MOUSSES AND GELS

The latest hair helpers are mousses and gels. They're superb for styling the new short, layered cuts and adding body to blunt-cut hair, particularly if it's fine-textured, limp or flyaway. They'll leave your hair soft and shiny, never stiff or sticky like old-fashioned setting lotions. Men often like using mousses and gels, too—they're much easier to apply and more natural looking than old-fashioned hair cremes.

Mousse is a light, airy foam that looks like shaving cream and comes in an aerosol can. You can buy mousse in "regular," "extra body" and "conditioning" formulas. Gels are clear and watery and come in tubes. They have a little more holding power than mousse. Use either mousse or gel by combing it into your hair after shampooing. Then you can style your hair using a brush and a blow-dryer or simply sculpt and contour the hair with your fingers. When applied before blow-drying, mousse or gel will help you control and direct the hair.

If you notice your scalp flaking after using a certain brand of mousse, switch to one that's alcohol-free or to a gel. A large amount of alcohol can sometimes irritate the scalp. The ingredients list on the package label will tell you whether or not the product contains very much alcohol.

Classic Blow-Drying Technique

The best way to add volume to the hair and give it a polished finish is by blow-drying. Anyone can learn to master the basic blow-drying technique. The steps are similar to those you'll follow when cutting the hair. The instructions below are for blunt-cut or layered hair that's straight or has a very slight wave. To style wavy to curly hair, you'd use your fingers and a diffuser (see "Styling Tips" on page 68).

1. Apply a little mousse or gel to your hair for more holding power.
2. Begin by making a center part from the top of the crown down to the base of the neck. You're going to blow-dry the hair in horizontal sections on each side of the part. Comb down a 1-inch-thick section of hair on one side. Pin up the hair above it with a large, thin metal clip so you can work with one section of hair at a time. Now place the brush under the 1-inch

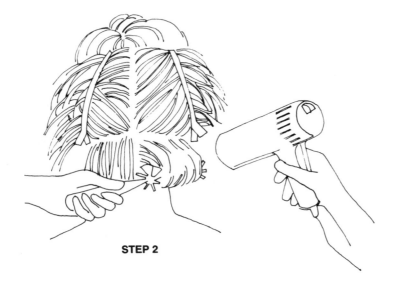

STEP 2

section and roll the ends of the hair under the brush twice. Holding the hair taut in the brush, switch on the blower and move it up and down from the roots to the ends of the hair for several seconds.
3. Take down a 1-inch section on the opposite side of the part. Clip the hair above it aside. Roll it under the brush and dry from top to bottom.
4. Keep drying 1-inch sections of hair on each side of the part all the way up to the crown.

5. Next do the sides, starting from the bottom and drying the hair section by section up to the part. While drying each section, clip up the hair above it. If your hair is layered, roll the side sections back away from the face and blow them dry.

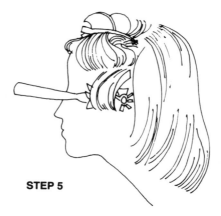

STEP 5

6. If you want straight bangs, roll them under the brush and blow them dry moving the blow-dryer back and forth. For side-swept bangs, roll the hair back away from the face and blow it dry from the roots up for more lift.

QUICKIE BLOW-DRY

If you don't have the time to do the basic blow-dry, there is a shortcut you can take. Simply brush all your hair forward over your face. Then blow it dry from the bottom up, constantly brushing your hair forward. Keep the dryer in constant motion until your hair is about 85 percent dry. For a smooth finish, roll the top layer of hair section by section around a styling brush and blow-dry for a few seconds. Then, roll the ends of the hair around the brush and blow-dry to turn them under.

BLOW-DRYING TIPS

• Never blow-dry hair when it's soaking wet. Towel dry it first to remove excess moisture. This way, your hair will dry faster. And the more quickly your hair dries, the easier it will be to get it to fall into line. When you rework the hair over and over again, it may lose body and become hard to manage.
• Stop blow-drying hair before it's completely dry. If you dry your hair completely it may become flyaway. You can also damage it by drying it too thoroughly too often.
• To avoid damaging your hair, always use the warm (not the hot)

setting and hold the dryer about 6 to 8 inches away from your hair. Also make sure to keep the blower in constant motion. Stylists at the salon often take a shortcut when blow-drying the hair. You may have noticed that your hairdresser directs a hot blast of air very close to a section of hair. This really isn't good for the hair, so don't do it at home. It won't hurt your hair if you do it every once in a while, but on a regular basis, you can dry out and damage it.

- If you want a smooth texture, style the hair with a brush. To enhance waves or curls, use your hands.

- If a section of hair gets tangled up in a round plastic brush, don't pull or tear at the hair; you could break it. To remove hair from the brush, gently pluck out pieces of it close to the roots until you free the whole section. Avoid overdrying fine hair. It might collect static electricity and become flyaway. To combat static, mist your hair with water and then work in a little mousse or gel.

- If you have a layered style and the hair at the top of the head looks flat after you're finished blow-drying, it's because the layers aren't short enough. Styling gel, however, can help give your hair a little more volume until you cut it.

SETTING UP SHOP 2

$\mathbf{A}$ well-lit bathroom with a large mirror is usually the best place for haircutting. You can easily sweep up snippings and can place your tools on the vanity next to the sink. If you don't have a vanity in your bathroom, line up tools on a shelf or set up a small table right next to you. A portable table on wheels that you can roll into the bathroom during haircutting is ideal.

Assemble Your Tools

When it comes to haircutting, organization counts. You'll want to have all your tools ready and within hand's reach before you start cutting. If you have to search around for clips and other items during the middle of a haircut, you won't be able to concentrate on what you're doing.

It matters what type of tools you use. A pair of household scissors, for instance, won't work for haircutting. They're too heavy and hard to handle and don't have a sharp enough cutting edge. To cut the hair well, you need a small collection of professional tools—the same kind that hairstylists use in the salon. You can pick them up inexpensively at a beauty or household supply store or at the drugstore. A good set of tools is a small investment to make if you'll be cutting your own hair on a regular basis. Following is a list of the items you'll need. You may already have some of them on hand.

Plastic Comb You'll want a slim, lightweight comb about 6 inches long and ½ inch wide. It's the perfect length, width and weight for haircutting. It will glide through the hair smoothly and help you pick up the right amount of hair when cutting. Because it's light as a feather, you'll find it extremely easy to work with.

Scissors A pair of professional haircutting scissors is your most important tool. Five-inch-long stainless steel scissors from a beauty supply store are best. They fit into the hand easily, allowing you to get a good firm grip. Pro scissors are much sharper than regular household scissors and will help you cut the

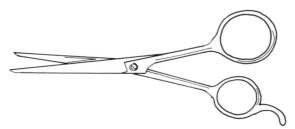

hair evenly. In addition, the stainless steel won't rust. Pro scissors come in greater lengths, but size has nothing to do with precision cutting. Large scissors can be awkward to handle.

Hair Clips Buy a package of long thin metal clips. Clipping up the hair you're not cutting will help you create precise partings— the key to good haircutting technique. Plus, you'll have a clear, unobstructed view of the section of hair you're working on.

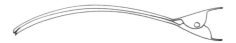

Clips should be sturdy and clasp the hair securely; they shouldn't slip out or let stray hairs escape. If pieces of hair fall down into the section you're working on, you won't get accurate results. You can also use fasteners that look like giant paper clips. Do not substitute bobby pins or small hair clips. They won't keep the hair secure and will make it more difficult to part the hair cleanly.

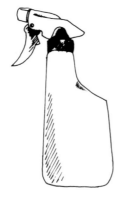

Mister You're going to need a plastic spray bottle filled with water to keep the hair damp throughout a haircut. If a section of hair dries, spritz it with the mister to instantly rewet it. Misting the hair is much faster and easier than wetting it with a comb dipped in water.

Towel   Have a bath-size towel nearby to dry the hair and wrap it up after washing it.

Mirror   In addition to a large mirror facing you, you'll need an extra mirror to see the back of your head. An adjustable mirror attached to a retractable, swing-out arm will give you the clearest view. You can position the handle to the back or side of your head. And you can adjust the mirror upward or downward. This way you'll be able to see your head at any angle. You can buy this type of mirror in a housewares store or in the home furnishings department of a hardware store.

Or you might have a big mirror around the house that you can use for haircutting. A full-length mirror set up behind you, for instance, would also work.

Cape   This is an optional item. If you're cutting long hair, it's not necessary at all. You'll want to keep the back and shoulders uncovered during haircutting to judge the length correctly. If you're cutting short hair, however, you might want to wear a cape to catch the snippings. A cape might also be more comfortable for kids. If you don't use a cape, wear an old top without a collar that leaves the back of the neck fully exposed. A collar conceals the neckline and gets in the way of cutting.

Fifteen Pro Tips

To get the best possible results you have to follow a few basic haircutting principles. Here are the techinques the pros use to cut the hair with precision.

1. Always start out with freshly washed hair. When it's clean and wet, your hair will be easier to control and you'll be able to cut it more accurately. If your hair dries out during a cut, rewet it with a plastic spray bottle. (Bangs are the only exception to this rule. You cut them dry to make sure they don't come out too short.)

2. Make clean, even partings—they're essential for a professional-looking haircut. One basic part you'll be using throughout the book is a diagonal one. You may want to practice parting the hair before you actually start cutting it so you can section it off quickly and neatly. Here's how it's done:

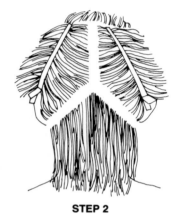

STEP 2

Part the hair in back from crown to nape. Then starting on one side, part off a 1-inch-thick section of hair on a diagonal angle toward the earlobe. Next, separate a diagonal section of hair the same size on the opposite side of the center. Now comb both sections together straight down against the nape of the neck. The hair should ressemble a triangular wedge or inverted V. Clip the hair above the diagonal partings up and out of the way. It will make it much easier to cut the hair precisely.

3. Get the handwork down pat. It's important to hold the scissors correctly. Hold them in your most dextrous hand. Slip your thumb through the top loop of the scissors and your ring finger through the bottom loop. Place your pinky under the bottom loop of the scissors to balance it. When you're cutting, the

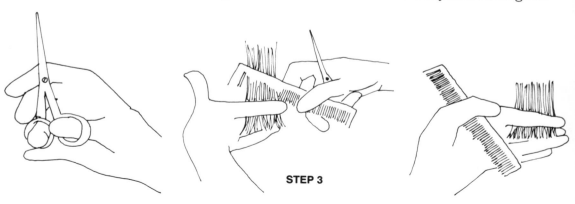

STEP 3

scissors always stay in the same hand, but you'll switch the comb from one hand to the other. Here's how this maneuver works: while you're parting the hair with the comb, hold the scissors in the crook of the same hand between thumb and index finger with the tips facing upward. When you're ready to cut the hair, transfer the comb to your opposite hand and hold it between your thumb and index finger. After you've practiced these motions, you'll be able to perform them smoothly.

4. Cut the hair about ½ inch longer than you want it to be. It will shrink when dry. If your hair is extremely curly, allow 1 inch for shrinkage.

5. Sit or stand up straight when cutting your own hair. Hold your head still and tilt it slightly in the opposite direction from which you're cutting. This will pull the hair taut so you can cut it perfectly straight. The same applies if you're cutting someone else's hair. Make sure that the person's posture is erect through-out the entire cut and that he or she provides a little resistance as you're cutting.

6. Keep in mind that the first piece of hair you cut in a section will be your guide for cutting the rest of the hair in that section. Never guess about how much hair you should cut off. Always refer back to the first piece. All of the hair in the same section should match it.

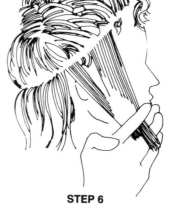

STEP 6

7. Use points on the body to help you during haircutting. The bones of the spine, for instance, can aid you in judging where to begin cutting the bottom line in back. The tips of the eyebrows can serve as markers for the width of bangs or where to start angling the hair for a layered cut. You can even use your thumbs to measure how much hair you're taking off. From the tip of the thumb to the first joint is about 1 inch.

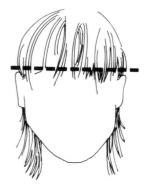

STEP 7

8. Hairdressers cut hair quickly, but that doesn't mean you have to. Take your time when doing a haircut. Cut the hair in small continuous snips, not big choppy bites.

9. For more control when doing a blunt cut, hold the hair down against the head with the side of your hand. You'll get a straighter line this way. When doing a layered cut, hold the hair out from the head on a diagonal angle at the nape, straight out at the center of the head and upward at the crown. Picking the hair up and out from the head creates a layered effect. Grasp sections of hair between your middle and index fingers to layer it and cut below your fingers.

10. When holding hair between your fingers, don't cut past the second joint of your index finger. You could accidentally nick the skin between the fingers.

11. There's a basic procedure to follow when cutting the hair in back. Make a 1-inch notch at the center of the nape to serve as your guideline for the length of the hair. Then cut the hair in ½-inch sections from the center to the left, and then from center to the right. As mentioned in step 6, each piece of hair you cut serves as the guide for the next. If you try to cut the hair all the way from one side of the head to the other, the length may come out uneven.

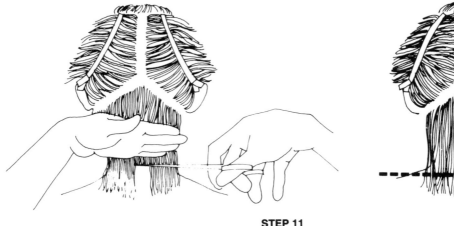 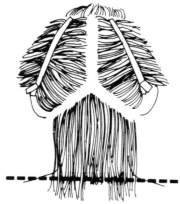

STEP 11

12. Always cut the hair in the direction in which it grows. Curly or wavy hair may curve to one side when you comb it down against the head. Don't try to force it to lie flat. Cut it as it falls naturally. Even a headful of straight hair may contain a lock or two that curves to one side. See the following section on cowlicks if you find an unruly piece of hair that grows in an entirely different direction from the rest.

13. To check the length of the hair, pinch sections on each side of the head between your thumb and index finger and pull them taut. The length should look even on each side.

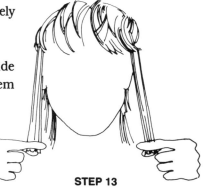

STEP 13

14. Take extra care to cut straight hair evenly. Mistakes will show more than on wavy or curly hair.

15. Trim your hair every six to eight weeks to maintain its shape.

Special Haircutting Problems— Licking That Cowlick

Before you cut your hair, take a look in the mirror to detect variations in the growth pattern. You may come across a quirky patch of hair, a cowlick, that has a direction all its own. You can reduce the effect of a cowlick by cutting and styling your hair to blend it in. Here are the various types of cowlicks and how to handle them.

Garden-Variety Cowlick   A tuft of hair that pops up and won't lie flat is the most common type of cowlick. You'll usually notice a cowlick like this along the hairline in the center of the forehead or slightly off to one side. They're most visible on straight hair.

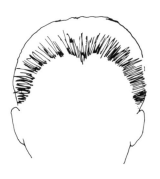

Part your hair through the center of the cowlick or slightly to the side of it so it falls into soft waves on each side of your forehead. You'll have to experiment with various part lines until you find the place where the cowlick divides naturally. For a more dramatic look, you can part your hair on the far side of the cowlick and sweep all the hair over the cowlick to the opposite side, holding it in place with a little gel. Cut each piece of the hair in the cowlick in the direction in which it grows.

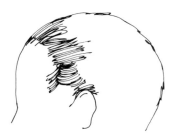

Widow's Peak A V-shaped cowlick at the center of the forehead is a widow's peak. The hair grows in an upward direction. You can blend a widow's peak into your hair to give it natural height. Make a side part and comb your hair over the peak. Use a dab of gel to hold the hair in place. Avoid a center part—the widow's peak will sprout out on each side of it. Don't cut the widow's peak any shorter than 1 inch. If you do, it will stick straight up.

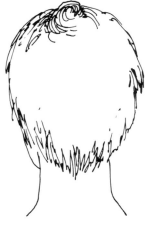

Pinwheel This is a swirl of hair that jumps up at the back of the crown, slightly to one side. It's very important to cut the hair in this type of cowlick in the direction in which it grows. Pull out each piece of hair in the pinwheel cowlick and cut it to conform to the natural growth pattern. If you cut it off in one big clump, pieces of the cowlick will stick up. When layering the hair short, leave a pinwheel cowlick about ¼ inch longer than the rest of the hair to prevent it from sticking up. You can also use a little gel to hold it down.

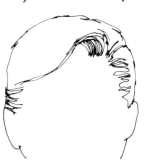

Curlicue If you have wavy or curly hair, you might find a cowlick that grows over the temple in two different directions: the hair along the hairline goes downward onto the face and the piece above it arcs backward. There are two ways to deal with this type of cowlick: you can use gel to direct it back away from the face or trim the piece growing forward close to the hairline so that it lies flat.

Precut Procedures

You'll be able to give yourself or someone else a pro cut if you prepare the hair properly before you begin cutting. Following are all the steps: don't skip any of them.

1. Wash your hair, gently massaging the shampoo into the scalp and working it out to the ends of the hair. Then rinse the hair thoroughly.
2. Apply the conditioner of your choice, leave it on for the time specified on the label, then rinse your hair well.
3. Pat your hair dry with a towel. Wrap the towel around your head like a turban for a few minutes to absorb excess moisture. Your hair should be wet but not dripping when you cut it.
4. Comb your hair, working from the ends up to the crown, using the wide-toothed side of the comb. Gently work out snarls section by section. Don't yank the hair—you could break it or pull it out by the roots.
5. Part your hair if the cut you're doing calls for it. Unless you have a cowlick, find your natural part line. Everyone has one. To locate yours, comb all the hair back off the face. Now tap your hair at the crown. Several separations will appear in the hair. Make a side or center part—whichever you prefer—along the strongest separation. Now follow the directions for the haircut you've selected.

PRECISION HAIRCUTTING 3

Ready to try out your skills? We've put together a roundup of terrific haircuts and styling tips for everyone. There's a cut here for every hair texture and taste.

It's best to ease into haircutting. You might want to begin by trying some of the styling tips ahead to get used to working with hair and to develop a feel for handling it. From styling you can progress to a trim or one of the simple styles such as cutting bangs or the one-step kids' cut. After you feel comfortable and confident about your abilities, try a major haircut. When cutting your own or someone else's hair for the first time, avoid making major changes. For instance, if your hair is long and you'd like a bob, try cutting it gradually shorter, month by month. That way, if you don't like it, you won't have to wait months for your hair to grow out. You might also discover the perfect cutoff point—the length at which your hair looks its best and is easiest to manage. If you have a good eye for design and a steady hand, you can probably do most of the cuts yourself. For others, you'll find it easier if a friend cuts your hair for you.

If you are unhappy with your hair after you cut it, live with it for a few days. You may decide you love it. It's always difficult to get used to a new haircut. Kids may find it especially hard to adjust to a different look. A good rule of thumb is to avoid cutting your own or anyone else's hair on impulse or when you're feeling below par. Think positively and psych yourself up for haircutting. Keep in mind that it's a methodical process. There's no guess-work involved if you follow our step-by-step instructions. And you can never lose your place because each piece of hair you cut will serve as a guide for the next piece. Before taking that first snip, it also helps to have the look you want to achieve crystallized in your mind. You may be surprised by the professional results you get. So go to it and get yourself a glamorous new look.

When you're constantly on the go, it's hard to give your hair the care and attention it needs. You may not have time to get it trimmed regularly, let alone pay a visit to the salon every week to have it styled. You may have worn your hair the same old way for years, simply because it's easy to handle. By learning to cut your own hair you can update your style and look perfectly polished. And the price is right! In the following pages, you'll find five fashionable cuts, plus tips on how to choose the one that flatters you most and goes with your natural hair texture.

CHOOSING A FLATTERING STYLE

When deciding how to style your hair, a professional haircutter will analyze your natural hair type and texture as well as your face shape and features. He or she will even take your height into consideration. You should take the same factors into account when trying to determine which style will be most flattering on you. You should never go with a style simply because you like it on someone else. It might not suit you at all. Here are some pointers on how to choose the style that will do the most for you and be easiest to manage.

Go With Your Hair Type and Texture

In addition to complementing your hair type—straight, wavy or curly—a haircut should go with your hair texture. If you checked the hair care chart on pages 20-21, you know whether your hair is fine or coarse. Or it may be somewhere in between: medium-bodied. If your hair has a fair amount of body, it has natural fullness and holds its shape well.

It's a mistake to try to force your hair into a shape it doesn't want to take. Blow-drying thick curly hair straight, for instance, takes a lot of time and your curls will come popping up anyway. By the same token, fine straight hair will look limper and flatter if you wear it long and layered. You have to be realistic about what your hair will and won't do. If your hair is straight and you're longing for a headful of curls, consider getting a perm. Here are the various types and textures of hair and the cuts that work best with them.

Wavy to very curly hair of all textures will look its fullest and fluffiest when layered. When worn all one length the natural curl in the hair is weighted down and looks shapeless or droopy. Layering releases the curl or wave and gives your hair volume and movement. If you have fine, very curly hair, wear it on the short side for the most body and control.

Fine straight hair will fall better and have more bounce and body when worn in a short blunt cut such as the bob. Or for a feathery look, wear it short and layered.

Coarse straight hair looks best in a long blunt cut. If you layer it, the steps will show. And if you cut it in very short layers, it will stick up.

Straight, medium-bodied hair will take to any style or length—long or short, layered or blunt-cut.

Analyze Your Face Shape

It's important to take stock of your facial shape and identify your best features before selecting a hairstyle. The right hairstyle can play up your assets and camouflage your flaws.

To determine your face shape, pull all your hair back, then take a look in the mirror. Here are the characteristics of the most common face shapes and the haircuts that flatter them.

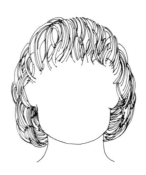

Square You have a broad forehead and jawline. A blunt cut below chin length with full, fluffy bangs will complement your strong bone structure.

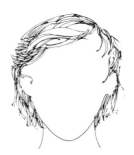

Heart Your face is widest at the forehead and tapers to a narrow chin. The cheekbones are usually highly visible. With your delicate features, you can carry off the shorter cuts well—an ear-length bob, for instance, or a layered cut that's quite short. A collarbone-length layered cut with soft side-swept bangs will also flatter your face shape and "fill out" your chin. Avoid off-the-face styles or thick straight bangs that emphasize your forehead.

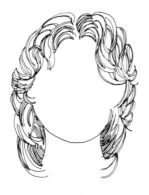

Round You have a very full face and the cheekbones aren't clearly defined. What you need is a hairstyle that creates the illusion of facial contours. Face-framing layers with bangs curving toward one side will sculpt angles into the face. Your hair should always be worn below chin length to make your face look longer and slimmer. Avoid a short bob or a long blunt cut parted down the center.

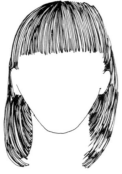

Diamond Your cheekbones are very prominent compared to your narrow forehead and chin. A shoulder-length blunt cut with a fringe of straight bangs will camouflage the fact that your face is widest in the center. It will make your forehead and chin look more evenly proportioned, too. A short curly layered cut will also do a lot for you: play up your cheekbones, hide your wide forehead and draw the eye up and away from your pointed chin.

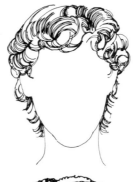

Long This type of face is thin and angular with a pointed chin. You want a hairstyle with height and width. A short layered cut with bangs spilling onto the forehead and fullness at the temples will make your face look wider. A collarbone-length layered cut that's very wavy or curly will also add softness and fullness to a long angular face. Steer clear of a long straight style that will make your face look more drawn out.

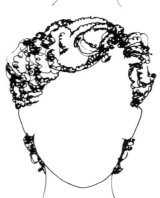

Oval An oval face is perfectly symmetrical with chiseled-looking cheekbones. If you're lucky enough to have a face this shape, you can wear your hair any way you like. All lengths and styles will look great on you.

Next, take note of your features. Bangs, for instance, can emphasize beautiful eyes or help to camouflage a high forehead. A large nose will look less prominent if you part your hair on the side rather than in the center and direct the hair away from the face. If you have a long thin neck, you won't want to wear your hair super short. Your neck will only look longer. On the other hand, if you have a short neck, you shouldn't wear your hair much longer than chin length or your neck will appear wider.

The Perfect Proportion

Your hairstyle should also be proportional to your height and build. Many professional hairstylists will ask you to stand up so they can get a better idea of how a style will relate to your body size.

In general, if you're petite, avoid long hair—it will only make you look shorter. A style that's chin to collarbone length will look best on you. On the other hand, if you're tall and large-boned, a very short cut will emphasize your size. Wear your hair collarbone length or longer. A sleek medium-length style is most flattering if you're overweight. Voluminous curls or very long hair will make you look heavier.

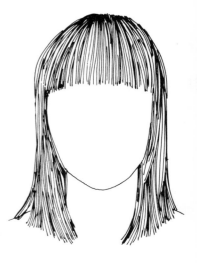

BLUNT CUTS

Technique: The long blunt cut and the bob both rely on the same basic method of haircutting. Each section of hair is combed horizontally over the previous one. The first section serves as a guideline for cutting the hair to the correct length.

LONG HAIR

Flaunt a headful of long shiny hair and you're sure to be noticed. Long beautiful hair is distinctive and can make you stand out from the crowd. Many models and actresses make long hair their trademark. Model Christie Brinkley, for instance, with her sunny blond hair, is the epitome of easy glamour. Actress

Catherine Deneuve's long pale blond hair contributes to her cool, classy beauty. Veronica Hamel (the fiery public defender, Joyce, on TV's *Hill Street Blues*) has a burnished brunette mane that adds a touch of femininity to the tough professional she portrays.

If your hair is straight and medium to thick, it can look just as fabulous as these celebrities'. You start with the most basic cut there is—the blunt cut. When cut cleanly, straight hair falls into a soft, swingy line. You decide on the cutoff point. You can wear your hair shoulder length or longer.

It's essential to trim long hair every six to eight weeks. Long hair is especially susceptible to split ends. Because the hair's natural oils are concentrated at the scalp, the ends of your hair may not receive enough moisture. As a result, they dry out and become split. Short wiry ends sticking up can sabotage the luxurious look of long hair. There's only one way to get rid of them and that's by cutting them off.

Don't attempt to do this cut on your own hair. It's impossible to reach around to the center of your back and cut your hair accurately. Enlist the help of a friend to do it for you. To add interest to long one-length hair, you might want to consider cutting bangs. They're a cinch to do with the instructions following the blunt cut.

INSTRUCTIONS

1. Wash and towel dry your hair. Comb it back off your face. If you're going to cut off 4 or more inches of hair, do a rough cut first to get rid of excess length. If not, skip this step and go on to step 2.

To do a rough cut, press the hair down in the center of the back using the flat of your hand and cut straight across about 2 inches below the desired length. Continue cutting over to the left side, then from center to far right. The hair doesn't have to be perfectly straight at this point. You can even out the line when you do the real cut. Just be sure to avoid cutting some sections of your hair considerably shorter than others.

2. Now you're ready to start the real cut. Part the hair down the center in back from crown to nape. Beginning 1 inch above the hairline, part the hair into two triangular sections and comb them together straight down against the nape. Clip the rest of the hair up so you have a clear view of the area you're working on.

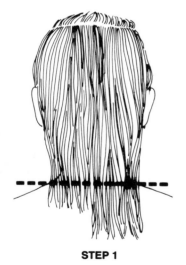

STEP 1

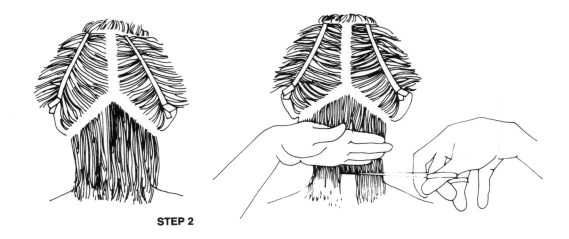

STEP 2

Press down the hair at the center of the nape with the flat of your hand and snip straight across until you've cut a 1-inch-wide section in the center. This notch will guide you in cutting an even bottom line. Continue cutting in 1/2-inch sections to the left side, pressing down each section of hair you're cutting as you go. Then return to the center and cut over to the far right side. The hair will come out perfectly even because you're always matching uncut hair to a section you've already cut beside it. *Tip:* When cutting the side sections of the hair nearest the ears, cut downward following the slope of the shoulders. This will prevent you from making the sides of the hair too short.

3. Part off two more diagonal sections 1 inch above the original partings. Clip the hair above them aside. Comb the new sections straight down over the hair you've just cut. Cut the hair to the same length as the section beneath it, snipping from center to left, then center to right.

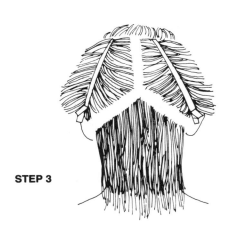

STEP 3

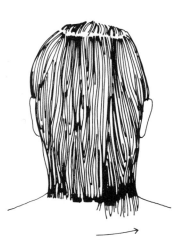

4. Keep parting off diagonal sections 1 inch above the previous partings and cutting from the center out to the sides. Rewet the hair if necessary so it lies completely flat against the back. When you reach the crown, you'll have one uncut section left over. Comb the hair straight down the back and cut off excess length to match the hair underneath it. At this point, you're halfway through the cut.

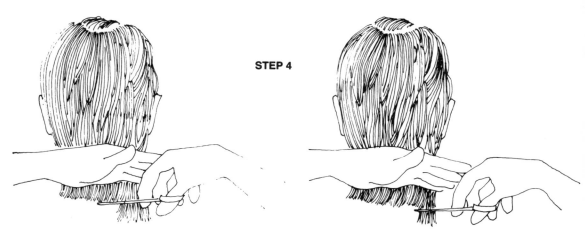

STEP 4

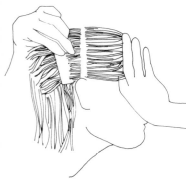

STEP 5

5. Next, you're going to match the sides of the hair to the hair you've already cut in back. To start, part the hair from ear to ear all the way across the crown.

6. Beginning on either side, make a second, horizontal part 1 inch above the ear and comb the hair straight down over the ear. Clip the hair above it aside. Now divide this section in half vertically, parting the hair in front of the ear. Let the section closest to the face fall free for the moment. You'll come back to it later. Comb a piece of hair from the back together with the section covering the ear. Holding the hair taut between your index and middle fingers and as close to the face as possible, cut the side section to the same length as the hair from the back. Snip from back to front, below your fingers. Then cut the remaining section of hair closest to the face to match the piece over the ear, again snipping from back to front. You've just created the bottom line for the side of your hair. You're going to cut all succeeding sections to the same length.

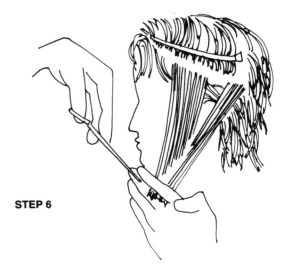

STEP 6

7. Separate the next horizontal section 1 inch above the first one and comb it in with the hair you've just cut. Cut it to the same length as the first section, snipping from front to back. Keep bringing down horizontal sections 1 inch above the previous parting and cutting to match the hair beneath them, until you run out of hair to cut.

8. Now go to the other side and repeat steps 6 and 7.

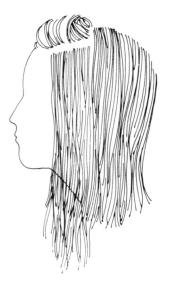

STEP 7

9. After you've finished both sides, check to see if they're even by grasping a section of hair on each side of your face between thumbnail and index finger. Pull the hair straight down to see if your thumbnails line up. If they don't, redo the horizontal sections until the hair is even.

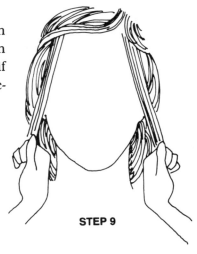

STEP 9

FOOLPROOF WAY TO CUT BANGS

At this stage, you might want to cut bangs to jazz up a basic blunt cut. The following steps result in bangs that you can wear forward or swept to one side. Or you can follow these directions to trim the bangs you already have. Doing your bangs is a minicut all by itself. Two of the most common reasons for botching up bangs are cutting them crooked or too short.

1. If you don't already have bangs, now is the time to do a rough cut. To trim bangs, skip this step and go on to step 2.

Spritz the hair above your forehead to wet it. Part the hair 1 inch back from the hairline and comb it forward over your face. You should be able to see through this sheet of hair. Next, section off the hair at the sides where you want the bangs to begin. A short fringe would start at the tip of each eyebrow. Deep, full bangs stretch from temple to temple.

Starting in the center of your forehead, hold a 1-inch section of hair between your middle and index fingers as close as possible to your face and cut at the tip of your nose. You'll want to leave your bangs long for the moment. Work your way over to the left side, cutting the hair in same-size sections; then cut from center to right.

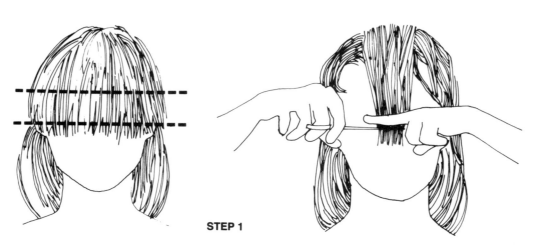

STEP 1

2. Let your bangs dry or blow them dry. Don't cut them wet because they may come out too short. For the final cut, divide the hair of the bangs into several layers. Part the hair 1/4 inch back from the hairline and comb it forward, flat against the forehead. Pin the rest of the hair back so you're working on one small section at a time.

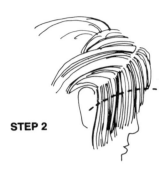

STEP 2

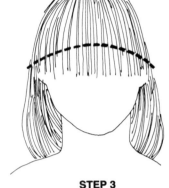

STEP 3

3. You'll want your bangs to be a little longer on the sides so they form a gentle curve following the contour of the forehead.

Starting on either side, where your bangs begin, press the hair down firmly with the flat of your hand and cut a 1-inch section of hair on a downward slant to right below the eyebrow. Go over to the other side and cut the same-size section on an angle toward the ear. The side sections will serve as your markers.

4. Now connect up the markers. Beginning on either side, press the hair down over the forehead and cut it in 1-inch sections just below the eyebrows to make sure it doesn't come out too short.

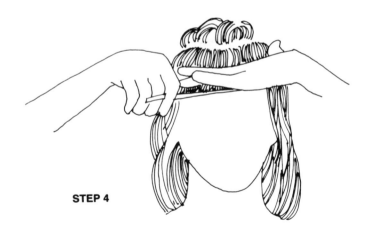

STEP 4

5. After you've finished the first layer of hair, comb down another ¼-inch layer. Cut to the same length and shape as the hair beneath, snipping from side to side.

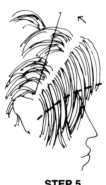

STEP 5

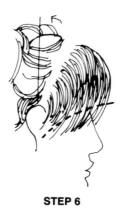

6. Keep combing down ¼-inch-thick layers and cutting them to match the bangs beneath them until you run out of hair to bring down.

Layered Bangs   If you'd like to wear your bangs brushed to one side, you might want to lightly layer them to give them more movement. To do this, you're going to cut your bangs in vertical sections from the part line to the tip of the eyebrow or the temple, wherever your bangs start.

Begin by parting off a section of hair 1 inch below the part. Hold it straight up between your thumb and index finger. You'll notice that this piece of hair will be short on each side and long in the middle. Cut the hair straight across from short point to short point.

Keep parting off your bangs in vertical sections 1 inch apart and snip off the long piece of hair in the center of each section. Now cut the bangs on the other side of the part the same way.

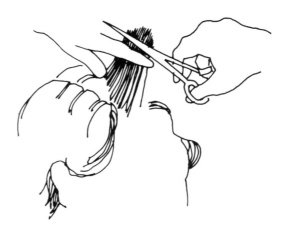

STYLING TIPS

Long hair allows many styling options. To give it a smooth, polished look, blow it dry following the directions on page 25. Or you can braid long hair, pull it back with combs or a headband, or sweep it up.

French Twist   If you'd like to make your hair look special for an evening out, try a French twist. It's a fast way to create a fancy style. All you'll need are some bobby pins and a long flat metal barrette.

To do, brush all the hair from the right side of the head over to the left, behind the ear. Put in the barrette vertically, slightly to the left of the center of your head to anchor the hair in place. Now grasp the ends of the hair at the nape and begin rolling them inward over the barrette to the center of the head. Pin the roll from underneath with small bobby pins. Keep rolling the hair inward and upward all the way to the crown, pinning in place as you go. At the crown, secure the inside of the roll to the scalp with a long bobby pin. If you have bangs, comb a little mousse or gel through them and fluff them up with your fingers for lift and volume.

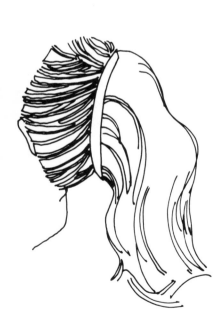
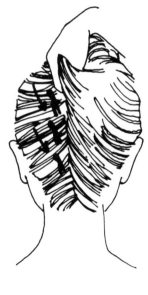

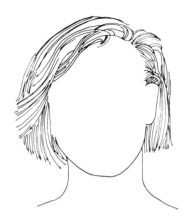

THE BOB

If you want a style that's basic but not boring, the bob can't be beat. This blunt cut is a revival of a style dating from the 1920s, with a modern twist.

The bob is easy to care for, yet polished enough for the office, and elegant enough for an evening out. It will even hold its shape during a strenuous workout. You can wear the bob anywhere from ear length to just below the chin, alone or with straight or side-swept bangs (see cutting how-tos on pages 48 to 50).

INSTRUCTIONS

1. Wash and towel dry the hair. Part it in the center or on the side, wherever you prefer.

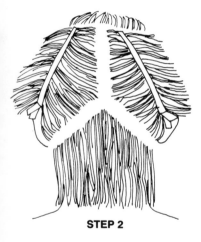

2. Now go around to the back and make a clean parting down the center of the head, from crown to nape. Part off two diagonal sections of hair on each side 1 inch above the hairline. Comb the hair straight down against the back of the neck. Clip the rest of the hair up out of the way.

STEP 2

3. With the back of your hand, press down the hair in the center back of your head. Snip straight across until you've cut off a 1-inch-wide section in the center. This notch will be your guideline to cutting the bottom of your hair evenly.

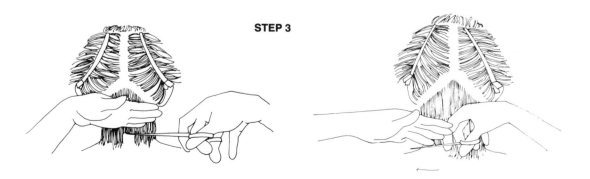

STEP 3

Continue cutting from center to left matching each piece against the guide, all the way over to the ear. Then cut from center to right, pressing the hair down firmly against the head as you go. You've now created the bottom line and will cut all the sections of your hair in back to the same length.

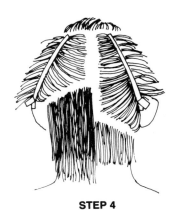

STEP 4

4. Separate two more diagonal sections 1 inch above the first partings and comb them straight down. You'll be able to see through the hair to your original line. Cut to the same length as the first section, from center to left, then center to right.

5. Continue parting off diagonal sections 1 inch apart and cutting to match the hair beneath them until you reach the crown. Make sure to keep the hair wet and press it down flat with the back of your hand to ensure an even line.

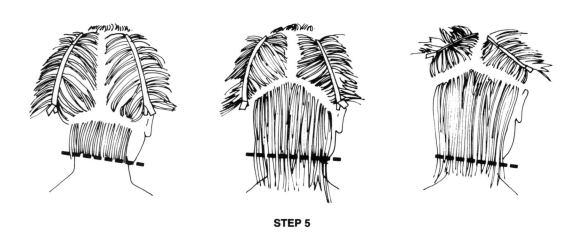

STEP 5

6. When you reach the crown, you'll have one uncut section left over. Comb it straight down the back of you head. Holding the hair flat against your head with your hand, cut to the same length as the hair beneath it.

7. Next, you're going to cut the sides of your hair to match the back. Part the hair from the center of each ear, all the way across the crown. Beginning on either side, part off a horizontal section of hair 1 inch above the ear. Clip the rest of the hair aside.

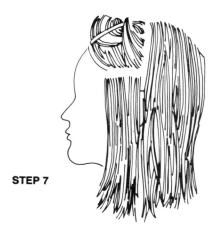

STEP 7

8. Divide the section of the hair in two by parting it down the middle in front of the ear. Pick up the section covering the ear, together with a piece of hair from behind the ear. Holding the hair taut between your middle and index fingers as close to the face as possible, cut the piece over the ear to the same length as the hair in back, snipping from back to front. Now take the section closest to the face and cut it to the same length as the piece over your ear. You've now created the bottom line for this side of your hair. You'll cut all succeeding sections to this length.

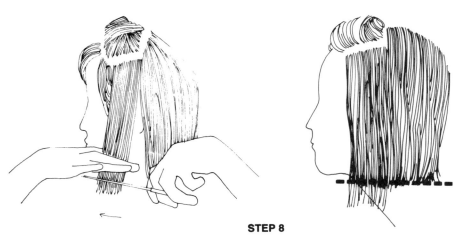

STEP 8

9. Part off another horizontal section 1 inch above the first parting. Cut it in two sections, first the hair over the ear, then the hair closest to the face, to the same length as the hair beneath it. Keep combing down same-size sections and cutting to match your original line until you reach the part.

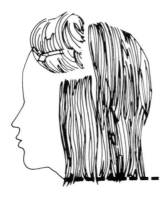 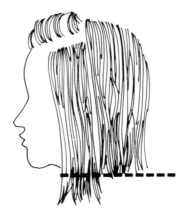

10. Now go on to the other side, on the opposite side of the part. Repeat the same steps, first combing down a horizontal section 1 inch above the ear. Divide it in two and cut the piece above the ear to match a piece from the back. Then cut off the hair closest to the face to the same length as the piece covering the ear. Continue combing down horizontal sections 1 inch apart and cutting them to match the sections beneath them.

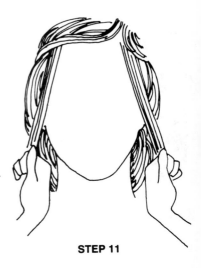

11. When you've finished cutting the sides of your hair, check to see if they're even by pinching a section of hair on each side of your face between thumb and forefinger. Pull the pieces of hair down taut and see if your thumbnails line up. If not, redo the side sections to straighten out the line.

STEP 11

12. If you want to add bangs, see page 48.

STYLING TIPS

The bob can be simple or sexy depending upon the way you style it. Blow-drying will give a bob the sleekest, shiniest look. If you prefer waves, apply mousse or styling gel and blow-dry your hair or let it air-dry as you scrunch it up with your fingers. To give a bob more bounce, consider giving yourself a "body wave" (see Chapter 4).

For evening, try slicking back one or both sides of your hair with gel. Or tie on a strip of black lace or a piece of metallic ribbon in gleaming gold or silver lamé.

LAYERED CUTS

Technique: The basic method for layering long and short hair is the same. Pieces of hair are combed out horizontally from the head together with a partial layer from a previously cut section. The hair is then cut to the length of the short piece.

LONG HAIR

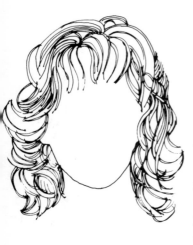

There's nothing more feminine than hair that falls in soft wispy layers around your face. Farah Fawcett first popularized the long layered look. Brooke Shields' voluminous waves are also based on a layered cut. Heather Locklear, who plays Sammi Jo on the TV series *Dynasty*, is another actress who flaunts long flattering layers.

Layering can be done on straight, wavy or curly textured hair. It gives the hair maximum volume. And it's so easy to care for that you can simply style it with your fingers after you wash it. You'll still be able to pull your hair back or wear it up. If you're concerned that it may be hard to grow out, we've included a grow-out cut on pages 75 to 80 to help you get through the transition in style.

If you're going to do your own hair, cut it to collarbone length—any longer than that and you won't be able to manage by yourself. If you want to wear your hair shoulder length or longer, you'll have to have a friend cut your hair for you. Another tip: If your hair is curly, it will shrink quite a bit when dry, so cut the hair 1 inch longer than you want it to be.

INSTRUCTIONS

1. Wash and towel dry your hair. Part it where you usually do, in the center or on the side. Now part it down the center from crown to nape. Separate a diagonal section 1 inch above the hairline on each side of the part and comb the sections together flat against the nape. If you're cutting your hair to collarbone length, feel for the bony knob at the top of your spine and begin cutting just below it.

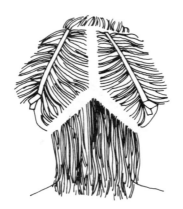

STEP 1

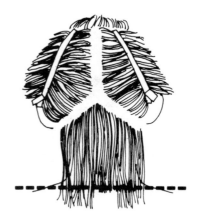

Holding the hair down against the head with the flat of your hand, begin cutting the hair in the center until you've snipped a 1-inch-wide section. This will serve as your guideline in creating an even bottom line. Continue cutting over to the left side, matching each piece to a guide piece, and pressing down the hair as you go. Then cut from center to right. When you're finished, you should have an even line across the nape of the neck.

2. Now go to the front of the head. Keep the hair you cut in back clipped up. You'll come back to it later. Comb down a layer of hair from part to ear, 1 inch back from the hairline. Pin the rest of the hair up. Starting next to the part, pull down a 1-inch-thick piece of hair over the forehead. Hold it taut between your index and middle fingers and cut to right beneath the eyebrow.

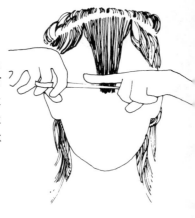

3. Now you're going to begin angling the sides. Establish an imaginary line in your mind by placing a comb against the side of your face angling from the hair you've cut in front to the hair you've cut in back.

To start, take a 1-inch-thick section of hair from over the temple between your thumb and index fingers. Pull it forward together with the piece of hair you cut from over the forehead and cut to the same length on an angle toward the earlobe. Refer back to page 43 for the basic principle of cutting a new section to the same length as a previously cut section.

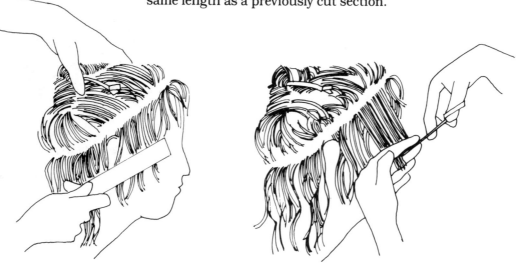

STEP 3

4. Take another same-size section, together with a piece of hair from above it, pull it forward and cut to conform to the same length and angle as the previous section. Keep picking up new sections, together with pieces you've already cut, and snip to match the preceding piece. When you reach the ear, comb a section of hair you've already cut in back together with the uncut hair over the ear. Hold the hair out on a diagonal and cut to identical length and angle.

5. Repeat steps 3 and 4 on the other side of the part.

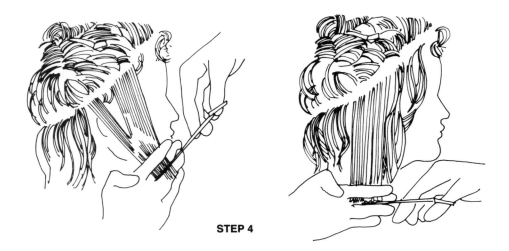

STEP 4

6. Next, finish cutting the hair in back of the head. Part off two more diagonal sections 1 inch above the first partings. Comb them over the hair you've already cut in back. To layer the hair, you're going to divide this large section into smaller, 1-inch-wide horizontal sections.

Starting in the center of the head, comb up a 1-inch-thick horizontal section of uncut hair, together with a partial layer of hair you've already cut from beneath it. (All you have to do is pick up a little of the hair from the old section. If you comb up the entire section of hair you've already cut, you'll have too much hair to work with at one time.) Hold the hair taut between your index and middle fingers and cut the top layer to the same length as the piece beneath it. Work your way over to the left ear, cutting same-size sections to the length of partial layers taken from underneath.

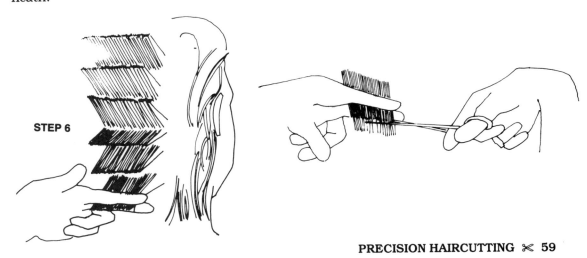

STEP 6

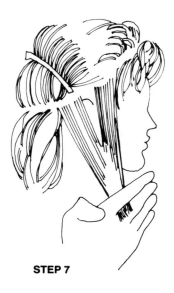

STEP 7

7. When you reach the ear, take a little bit of hair from in front of the ear together with the hair from in back of it. Hold this section out on a diagonal from the head and cut to the same length and angle.

8. Go back to the center of the head and cut the hair in 1-inch sections to the length of the hair underneath, all the way over to the right ear. Cut the section behind the ear to match a piece from the side over the ear.

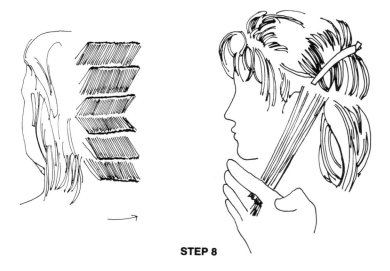

STEP 8

9. Work your way toward the crown, bringing down new diagonal sections, dividing them into smaller sections and cutting to match a partial layer of hair beneath them. You'll notice that you're cutting off larger pieces of hair as you get to the center of the head. Lift the hair up to cut it as you proceed upward. If small pieces of hair fall out of the comb as you pick up new sections, let them go. This is what creates the layered effect. Make sure to match up the hair in the sections closest to the ear with the angled hair on the side.

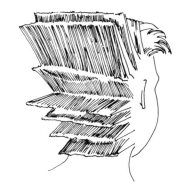

STEP 9

10. After you've cut the hair at the crown, go back to the side that you cut first. Comb down a layer of hair from part to ear, 2 inches back from the hairline, over the hair you've already angled. Starting at the part, comb a 1-inch-thick section of hair up vertically, together with a piece you first cut from over the forehead. Hold the hair taut and cut to the length of the short piece.

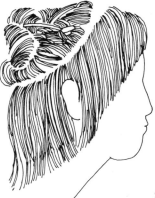
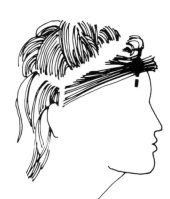

STEP 10

11. Comb up another vertical section, working in hair you cut above the temple. Hold the hair straight out from the head and cut to match the shortest point. Proceed down toward the ear, picking up new sections, together with pieces you've already cut, and snip to the same length. Always cut the hair to match the shortest point and hold it out in the direction in which it grows.

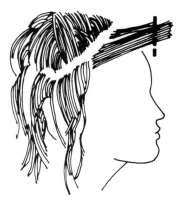

STEP 11

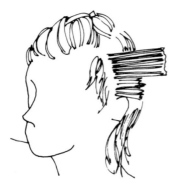

STEP 12

12. When you reach the section over the ear, comb it together with a piece of already cut hair from behind the ear. Pull this section straight out from the head and cut to the same length.

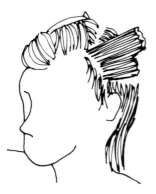

STEP 13

13. Comb down another layer of hair, 3 inches back from the hairline, from part to ear. Cut in 1-inch vertical sections with the hair from the layer below it. You're going to wind up with a triangle of hair that extends from the part back to the crown. Cut this last layer the way you did the others.

14. Repeat steps 10 through 12 on the opposite side of the part.

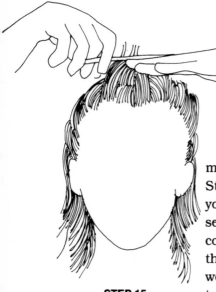

STEP 15

15. Check the hair all over the head to make sure you haven't missed any long pieces. Comb all the hair back off the face. Starting at the hairline in the center of the head and working your way down to the nape, comb up 1-inch-thick horizontal sections and cut off any long pieces. When you reach the nape, comb sections of hair upward to check them. Next, starting over the front hairline at the temple, comb hair up diagonally and work your way down to the nape. Check the hair over the other temple the same way.

STYLING TIPS

Let your hair air-dry or blow it dry with a diffuser while fluffing it up with your fingers. Here's how to get a full, voluminous look: work some mousse or gel through your hair. Using the fingers, pull the hair up and out from the roots and squeeze the waves or curls between your palms and fingertips until the hair is dry. Then, bend your head so your hair is hanging forward over your face and brush from nape to front.

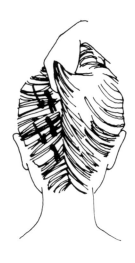

Evening Upsweep   If you'd like to give long, layered hair more impact for evening, wear it in a soft, sexy upsweep. Here are the how-tos:

You're going to form the hair into a modified French twist in back. It might take a little practice, but you'll get the hang of it after a few tries. Begin by brushing your hair back behind your ears. Now, grasp your hair in both hands at the center of the nape and start twisting it into a soft vertical roll. Pull the hair upward and keep twisting it all the way up to the crown, pinning it in place with small bobby pins or hairpins as you go.

You'll have some loose ends left at the crown. Tuck the ends under the top of the twist and pin in place with a bobby pin.

Now, using a little mousse or gel, lift the hair framing the face in the direction of the wave or curl to give it height and movement. If you like, spray lightly with hairspray to keep it in place.

SHORT HAIR

The latest trend for hair is toward short layered styles. Princess Di's soft, sleek style, for instance, starts with a short layered cut. Joan Collins (the wicked and ambitious Alexis Colby on *Dynasty*) has a curly layered style that's sexy and sophisticated. Today's crop of cuts differ from short styles popular in the past. Take the mod look of the 1960s, for example. To create it, the hair was cut on an exaggerated angle resulting in a style that looked severe and contrived. The new wave of short cuts is unique because for the first time the emphasis is on softness—short hair with ease that's built right into the cut. Now short layered hair is meant to look tousled and carefree, and altogether feminine.

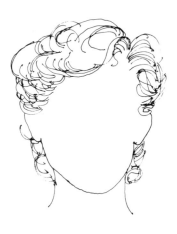

If you'd like to update your image or simply want a refreshing change from a conservative style, a short layered cut could be the answer. This type of cut is especially flattering for very curly, wiry hair. Also consider this kind of cut if you have practically no time

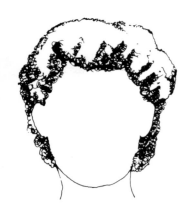

to spend on the care and styling of your hair. It's the easiest style of all to maintain. An unexpected advantage of a short layered cut is that your hair will stay its healthiest. Short hair isn't as susceptible to split ends as long hair because it's cut more frequently.

Cutting your hair short, however, is a major decision, so think about it carefully before you decide to do it. Yet short hair still offers you a variety of styling options. With the aid of mousse or gel you can comb the hair forward, back, up or down. In fact, short hair can look even more dramatic than long hair. See the styling tips on page 68. With a little experimentation, you'll find that short hair lends itself to a number of great looks.

INSTRUCTIONS

1. Wash and towel dry the hair. Part it in the center.

2. Pull down a section of hair on one side of the part, 1 inch back from the hairline. Holding it taut between your fingers, cut it straight across right below the eyebrow.

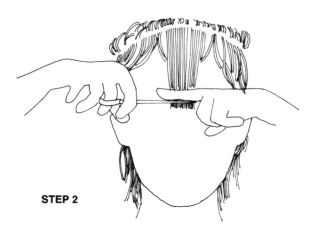

STEP 2

3. Now you're going to start angling the sides. Starting 1 inch back from the hairline, comb a layer of hair from temple to ear forward onto the side of the face. To visualize the angle before cutting, line up a comb on the side of the face and draw an imaginary line from the tip of the eyebrow to the center of the ear.

Take a section of hair from above the temple, together with a piece of hair you cut from above the forehead. Pull the hair out from the head and cut on a slant toward the ear, to the same length as the first piece.

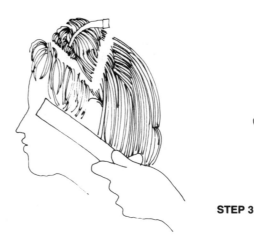
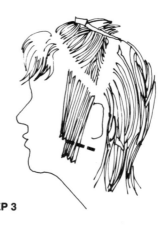

STEP 3

4. Pick up another section of hair, together with a piece from above it that you just cut. Snip to the same length and angle. Continue working your way down the side of the head to the center of the ear, cutting same-size sections conforming to this angle.

5. Repeat steps 2 through 4 on the opposite side of the part. Your hair will now frame your face in the front and on the sides.

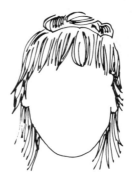

STEP 5

6. Now go back to the side where you started. Comb down a layer of hair from part to ear, 2 inches back from the hairline. You're going to begin cutting the hair in vertical sections. Starting next to the part, comb a 1-inch-thick section of hair straight up, together with a piece of the hair from the forehead that you've already cut. Holding the hair taut, cut it straight across to the same length as the short piece.

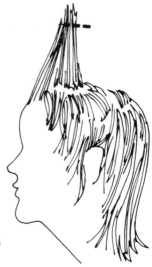

STEP 6

7. Comb up another vertical section below the one you just cut. Work in some hair from the section in front of it. Cut to match the shortest point. In this way, bangs will gradually be formed across the front of your head.

8. Work your way down to the ear, cutting the hair in vertical sections, always taking in pieces from the layer in front. You're forming progressively shorter layers as you move downward. When cutting, hold the hair out in the direction in which it grows—straight up at the top of the head, outward at the sides and on a downward angle when you reach the ear.

9. Repeat steps 6 to 8 on the other side of the part. You'll wind up with one last wedge of hair at the top of the head. Cut it the same way.

10. Now you're going to cut the back of your hair. Part it down the center from crown to nape. Separate two diagonal sections. Press the hair against the back of the neck firmly, using the flat of your hand. Cut the hair to the desired length, about 1 to 2 inches below the ear. Start in the center and cut a 1-inch section. Continue cutting to the left, then, using the first piece as a guide, from center to right. You've just formed the bottom line of your hair.

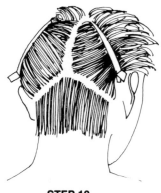

STEP 10

11. Next, you want to cut the side sections in back to conform to the same angle as the hair on the sides of your head. To do this, starting on either side, comb the hair over the ear straight down. Pull forward a section of hair from behind the ear to meet it and cut to the same length and angle as the hair above the ear. Do the same thing on the other side of the head.

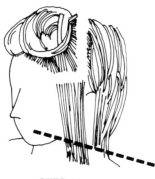

STEP 11

12. Part the hair again and bring down two more diagonal sections. Comb them in with the hair you've already cut. You're going to divide the hair in the large section into smaller 1-inch-wide pieces to layer it.

Starting in the center, comb up a horizontal section of hair, including a partial layer you already cut from beneath it. Pull the hair away from the head and cut the top layer to match the bottom piece. Work your way from center to left, then from center to far right, combing same-size sections together with pieces of hair from underneath. Snip them to the same length. When you reach the sides, make sure to cut on an angle that matches the sections above the ear.

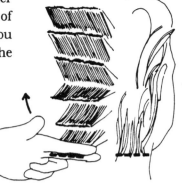

STEP 12

13. Keep combing down diagonal sections from each side of the part and dividing them into smaller sections containing a partial layer of hair you've already cut. Cut the top layer to match the hair underneath. As you work your way upward, you'll be taking off larger and larger pieces. Lift the hair up a bit and away from the head while you're cutting it. This is what creates the layered effect. When cutting the last sections at the crown, hold the hair straight up in the air to cut it.

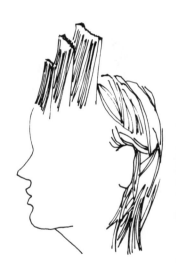

14. The last step is to check the hair on top of the head for any stray, long pieces you might have missed. Comb all the hair back off the face. Starting at the hairline, directly above the forehead, comb up a 1-inch-thick horizontal section of hair. If the piece is long in the center, cut off the excess. Keep working your way back to the crown, combing up horizontal sections and cutting any long pieces you find. The layers in back are so short it's not necessary to check them.

STEP 14

STYLING TIPS

You can style short layered hair many different ways using mousse or gel. If your hair is straight and you simply want more body, comb through some mousse or gel and blow it dry following the blow-dryer technique in Chapter 1. For maximum volume, back brush your hair after blow-drying. Bend your head and brush your hair forward and blow-dry from nape to front.

Let curly or wavy hair air-dry or blow it dry with a diffuser while you scrunch it between your palms and fingertips for more volume and texture. Set very curly, wiry hair on rollers to create softer curls.

There are also many special effects you can create. Work in some mousse or gel and experiment with these different looks:

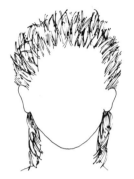

"SPIKED LOOK"

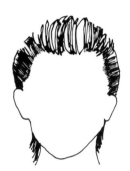

"WET LOOK"

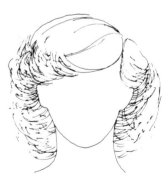

"PRINCESS DI LOOK"

- Slick your hair back behind your ears or comb one side forward and the other side behind your ear. Or pull the front section forward so it spills softly over your forehead.
- A spiked look can be glamorous for night. To create it, put a small amount of gel on the top of the head only. Then, section by section, lightly tease the hair with a comb or small brush for lots of height. Finish by applying a little more gel to the tips of the hair to hold it in place.
- For a wet look, comb gel through the hair after washing it and slick it all back off your face. Tousle or scrunch the hair over your forehead for more texture. This is an especially good style for hot summer days.
- If you, like Princess Di, have straight or wavy hair with a deep wave in the front, you can recreate her sleek style with ease. If not, you'll have to rely on setting gel or a curling iron to make your hair wave back.

  For the Princess Di look, start by partially blow-drying your hair 2 inches back from the hairline on the front and sides. Blow-dry back and away from your face. Separate hair into several sections and wrap them over and around a round styling brsh. Turn the handle of the brush twice to secure the hair and create a deep wave. Blow each section dry from roots to ends. Or you can use a curling wand to create a stronger curl. Wrap each section of hair over and around the wand and turn the handle one revolution.

To do the back, you simply blow-dry following the shape of the style, and turning the ends under.

THE MODERN CUT FOR WAVY TO CURLY HAIR

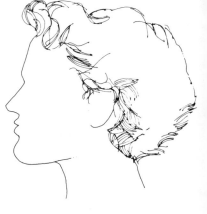

What makes the following cut so special is its shape. It's close-cropped at the nape and sides of the head and full in back. The hair is directed off the face in front and upward and outward in back. Result: a soft, pretty and very stylish look. This cut is for wavy to curly hair only. If you have straight hair and would like to try it, perm your hair first.

The cut uses two types of layers: horizontal and vertical. Both techniques are basically the same. The only difference between the two is the *direction* in which the hair is cut. The illustrations make this concept clear.

This cut is complicated, so don't try it unless you've mastered the basic haircutting techniques in this book. Instead, you might want to take these directions to a professional hairstylist and let him or her do the haircut.

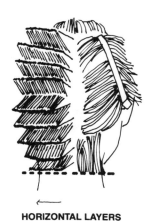

HORIZONTAL LAYERS

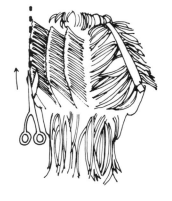

VERTICAL LAYERS

INSTRUCTIONS

1. Wash and towel dry the hair. Part it in the center from crown to nape. Comb down a diagonal section on each side of the part in back. Set the bottom line ¹/₂ to 1 inch below the ear. Holding hair down flat with the back of your hand, cut off a 1-inch wedge in the center to use as your guideline. Then, snipping ¹/₂-inch sections at a time, work your way out from the center to each end of the section. If any hair is growing below the hairline, trim it off. *Tip:* Curly or wavy hair may curve to one side when you comb it down against the head. Don't try to force it to lie flat. Instead, cut it in the direction in which it grows.

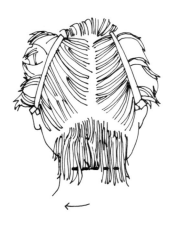 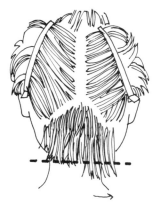 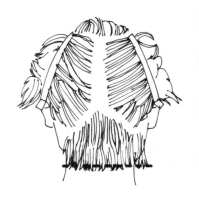

2. Comb down the next diagonal section 1 inch above the one you just cut. You're going to divide the hair in the large section into smaller 1-inch-thick horizontal pieces to cut it. Separate the first horizontal piece in the center of the head and work your way over to each ear, doing one side at a time. Comb each piece straight out at a right angle to the head. Comb in a little hair from the first layer you cut and cut to the length of the short piece.

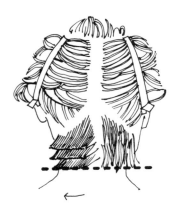 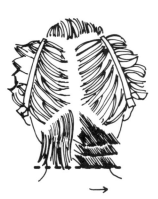

STEP 2

3. Continue layering the hair horizontally until you reach the bone a few inches from the bottom of the skull. At this point, you're going to make the layers longer. This step is very important because it will set the length of all the other layers in the back of the head. Separate another diagonal section of hair, 1 inch above the last one. Pick up a 1-inch-thick horizontal layer, pull it straight out from the head along with a piece from the layer beneath it and cut to the length of 1½ inches. Here's an

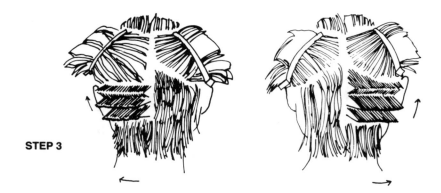

STEP 3

easy way to estimate length: from the end of the bottom layer, which is ½ inch long, measure down to the first joint of the thumb. This section of the finger is about 1 inch long. Continue cutting the rest of the hair in the large section, working your way out from the center to the sides.

4. Comb down another wedge of hair 1 inch above the one you just cut. Now begin layering the hair **vertically** in 1-inch-thick sections, starting at the center part. Match the top layer to the 1½-inch-long layer beneath it. Pull the hair straight away from the head to cut.

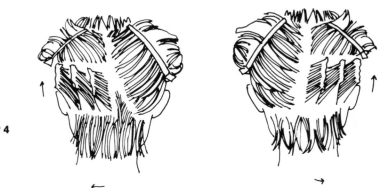

STEP 4

5. Repeat vertical layering all the way up to the crown. At the crown, hold layers out diagonally from the head.

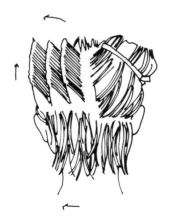
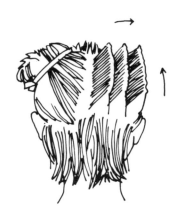

STEP 5

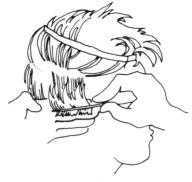

6. Comb down a 1-inch-thick horizontal section over one ear. Comb in some hair from behind the ear with the hair over the ear. Pull hair straight down and cut to the length of the short piece. The hair will be very short—¹/₂ to 1 inch long.

7. Comb down another horizontal section over the ear, together with the hair you just cut. Flip up the top layer so you can see the bottom one and cut to the length of the shortest piece.

8. Continue layering the hair over the ear, horizontally. Stop when you're about 1 inch above the ear. Snip off straggly hairs around sideburns for soft shaping or cut them on a sharp geometric angle. Also cut off any hair over the ear.

STEP 7

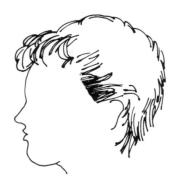
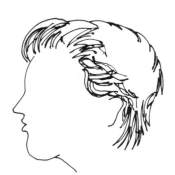

STEP 8

9. Repeat steps 6 to 8 on the opposite side of the part.

10. Part off a 1-inch-thick section of hair across the front of the head, stopping 2 inches above the ear on each side. Comb the hair straight down over the forehead. Pick up a section of hair in the center of the forehead, hold it straight down and cut to ½ inch below the brow.

11. Pull a section of hair from over one temple backward to meet the short hair over the ear and cut off any long pieces. Do the same thing with the hair over the opposite temple.

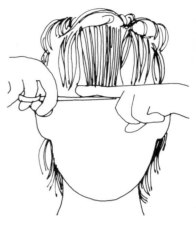

STEP 10

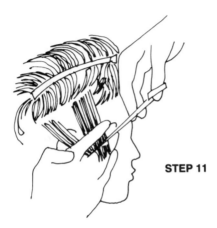

STEP 11

12. Comb down another 1-inch-thick horizontal section over the forehead. Starting at the center of the head, comb a vertical section of hair straight up together with a piece from the first layer over the forehead. Use the lower piece as a guide and cut the longer hair to match the short piece.

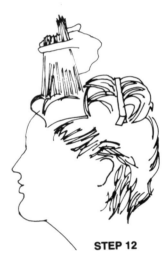

STEP 12

13. Comb up a vertical section of hair below the one you just cut. Comb in a piece from the first layer over the forehead and cut to match the short piece. Work your way down the head, layering the hair vertically. Stop 2 inches above the ear, then go back to the center and layer the hair vertically on the other side in the same way.

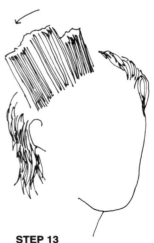

STEP 13

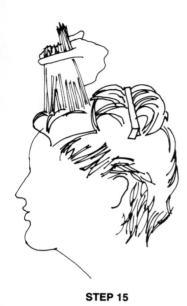

STEP 15

14. Work your way from the center of the head back toward the crown, parting off 1-inch-thick horizontal sections and layering them vertically.

15. When you reach the crown, comb vertical layers straight up together with pieces of hair from the last layer you cut in back. Cut to the length of the short piece from the front. This is how to blend the layers from the front with the layers from the back.

16. The last step is to check for any long hairs you might have missed during layering. Start combing up horizontal sections in the center of the head, working your way from forehead to nape. Hold the hair straight up and cut off any long pieces. As you work your way down the back of the head, pull hair in the direction in which it grows. When you reach the bottom of the head, comb hair upward to check it. Next check the hair over the temples. Comb it up diagonally starting at the front hairline and work your way down to the nape on each side.

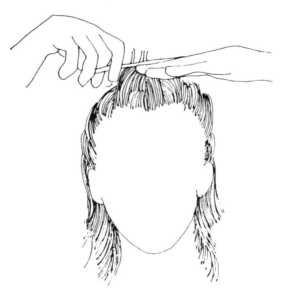

Styling Tip: Work some gel through freshly shampooed or dampened hair. Now style your hair with your fingers. Pull it straight up in front and on top of the head. In back, pull the hair upward and outward.

GROWING OUT YOUR HAIR—HOW TO GO FROM LAYERED TO ALL ONE LENGTH

Your hair doesn't have to look shapeless and straggly while you're trying to grow out a layered cut. You can keep it looking smooth, neat and stylish. The trick is to let the layers grow while you keep trimming the length. After a while, the layers will catch up to the length. You may be able to grow out long, layered hair in three to four months if you're willing to go to a short blunt-cut style. It may take up to a year to even out short layered hair. Don't try to grow out your bangs at the same time as the layers—wait until your hair is one length again. If you don't, your hair will tend to look ragged and you might be tempted to get it layered all over again. Take the growing-out process step by step and it will be much easier.

Trim your hair regularly, every six weeks, and it will grow out faster. The grow-out cut is for straight to wavy hair. Curly hair should never be worn all one length.

INSTRUCTIONS

1. Wash and towel dry hair. Part it down the center from crown to nape. Separate a diagonal wedge of hair in back of the head. Clip the rest of your hair up and out of the way. Set the bottom line 1 inch below your hairline in the back. Your hair will come out about even with your jawbone. Begin by cutting a 1-inch section in the center of the wedge. Use the back of your hand to hold the hair flat against the head. Now cut the hair to the left to match the center piece. Then snip to the right, using the center piece as a guide.

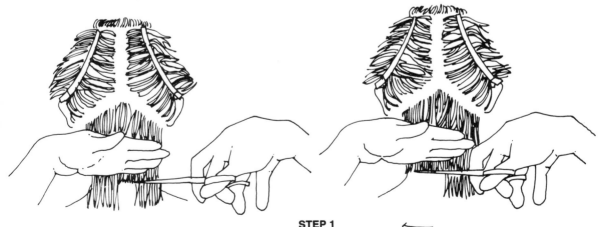

STEP 1

2. Separate another diagonal wedge of hair and comb it down over the layer you just cut. Trim off any hair that hangs below the bottom line you set, cutting the hair from the center out to the sides.

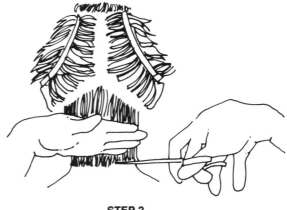

STEP 2

3. Work your way up the back of the head, bringing down wedges of hair. Comb over the previous layer you cut and trim to equal length. As you work your way up the head toward the crown, the layers will get shorter.

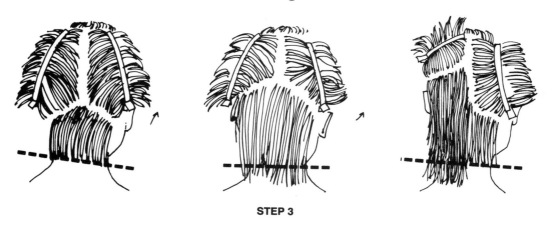

STEP 3

4. When you comb down a wedge of hair that's shorter than the bottom line, cut the hair like this: pick up a ½-inch-thick piece of hair from the center of the wedge and comb it out vertically from the head. Hold the piece of hair tautly between your fingers and cut off any long strands you find. The stray strands are often in the center of a section of hair, so cut the section from short point to short point. Work your way from

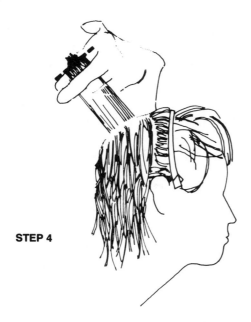

STEP 4

center to left and then right, separating ½-inch-thick vertical sections of hair and evening them out. You're cleaning up the layers so your hair will grow out evenly.

5. When you reach the crown, part your hair where you usually do. Then make another part, from ear to ear, and clip up the hair. You're going to cut the rest of the hair in three 1-inch sections. To start, comb down 1 inch of hair all around the face and over the forehead. This will help you see how long the layers are.

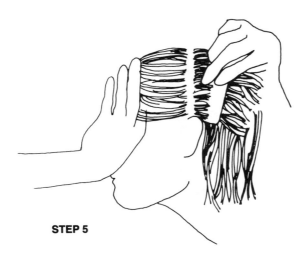

STEP 5

6. If the hair over the ear is longer than the hair you cut in back, cut it to match the length of the bottom line. If it's shorter than the hair in back, skip this step. To match the back with the sides, pull a section of hair forward from the back to meet a piece from over the ear. Hold the two pieces between your middle and index fingers and cut to the same length.

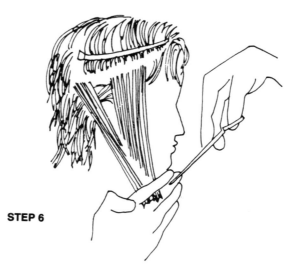

STEP 6

7. Now you're going to neaten the angle of your hair so it won't look straggly or ragged as it grows out. Comb out a ½-inch vertical section of hair from above one ear, and hold it diagonally away from the head. Trim off ¼ inch and any long, stray pieces that you find. Separate another ½-inch-thick vertical piece of hair above the one you just cut together with a small piece from the previous section and trim to the same length. Proceed cutting vertical layers up the side of the head until you've cut the hair over the temple the same way.

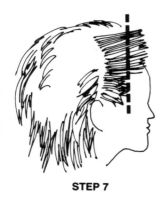

STEP 7

8. Cut the bangs on that side to brow level. Hold straight down between your fingers and snip evenly.

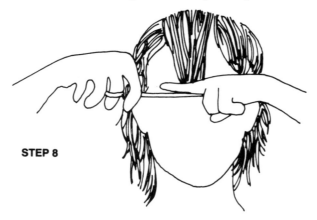

STEP 8

9. Repeat steps 6 and 7 on the opposite side. When you reach the forehead, line up the uncut bangs with the section you already cut on the other side, and trim them to the same length.

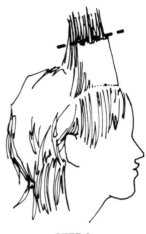

STEP 9

10. After you've done both sides, comb down the next 1-inch section of hair from ear to part. Match the hair in the back to the hair on the side by pulling a piece of hair from behind the ear to meet the section over the ear. Then cut to the same length.

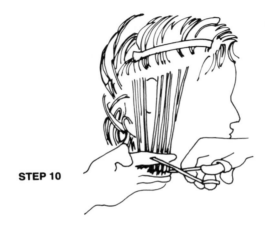

STEP 10

11. Now begin sectioning the hair vertically. Starting over the ear, comb a ½-inch-thick section of hair vertically out from the head, mix in a little hair from the layer underneath and cut off

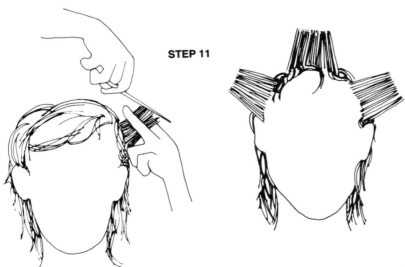

STEP 11

any long pieces. Work your way up from the ear to the temple to the part line. If the vertical sections look even when you pull them away from the head, don't cut off any hair. When you reach the top of the head, pull the hair straight up, like spokes on a wheel. Repeat this process on the opposite side of the part: beginning by combing down a 1-inch section of hair from ear to part, then dividing into smaller vertical pieces.

12. Go back to the side you started on. Bring down the last 1-inch-thick section of hair from ear to part. Begin sectioning the hair vertically, moving up the side of the head from ear to temple. Repeat on the opposite side of the part.

Haircutting and Styling for Men

If you're like most men, you're probably in the habit of going to the barbershop to get your hair cut. The style is basic and the price is right. But chances are, the cut is not very distinctive and may be downright boring. You keep going back though, out of habit or because you don't want to devote a lot of time to caring for your hair. You can, however, have great-looking hair without much effort. If you're plagued by a hair problem such as hard-to-tame texture or an unruly cowlick, a good haircut will cure the problem. You may also be concerned about hair loss. If you are, you're not alone. It's one of the most common hair woes among men of all ages. You'll be happy to know there are cutting techniques that will help disguise a balding pate.

There's more emphasis than ever today on presenting the right image for both women and men, so it's worthwhile to pay a little attention to your hair. We've provided everything you need to know to keep your hair in top form—cuts, styling tips, camouflage tricks, plus how-tos for trimming a mustache and beard. You may discover you're quite handy with a pair of scissors. If so, you can take over as the family's haircutter.

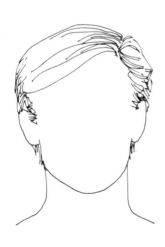

MEN'S LAYERED CUT

This cut looks good on any man. It's got class and dash and is therefore a vast improvement over the average barbershop cut. Whether you're a busy professional or a more rugged type, you'll like the clean-cut good looks of the layered cut. It's similar to the layered cut for women, with some modifications. For that reason, we've abbreviated the instructions here, so you may want to review the short layered cut on pages 64 to 67 before you begin.

INSTRUCTIONS

1. Wash and towel dry the hair. Part it on the side or in the center, depending on your preference.

2. Separate a section of hair above the forehead, next to one side of the part, 1 inch back from the hairline. Holding the hair straight down between your index and forefinger, cut it to 1½ inches long. This piece will set the length for the hair on the top and sides of the head.

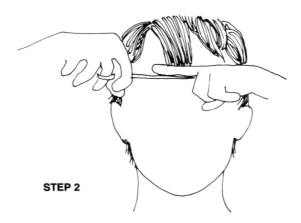

STEP 2

3. On the same side, part off a section of hair from temple to ear and comb it forward onto the face. Pick up a section of hair 1 inch thick from above the temple along with a little piece of hair from over the forehead. Hold the hair out diagonally from the head and cut on an angle toward the ear to the length of the first piece.

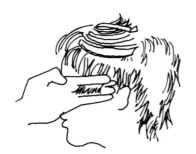
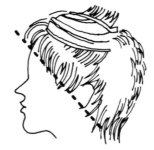

STEP 3

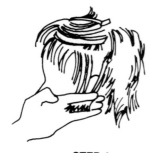

STEP 4

4. Work your way down the side of the head, cutting new sections of hair to conform to the same angle as the preceding pieces.

5. Repeat steps 2 through 4 on the opposite side of the part.

6. Go back to the side where you began. Separate a section of hair from part to ear, 2 inches back from the hairline. Beginning next to the part, comb a 1-inch-thick section of hair straight up together with a little piece of hair from the first section you cut over the forehead. Holding the hair taut, cut it straight across to the same length as the short piece.

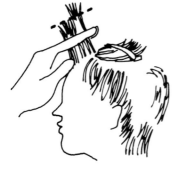

STEP 6

7. Go down 1 inch and comb up another vertical section together with a partial layer from the section preceding it. Cut to an equal length.

8. Continue cutting the hair in vertical sections containing small pieces from the layer preceding until you reach the ear. Make sure to hold the hair out from the head in the direction in which it grows.

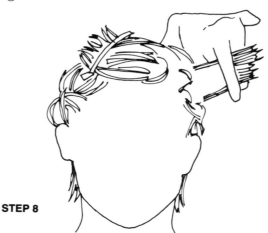

STEP 8

9. Repeat steps 6 through 8 on the opposite side.

10. Go to the back of the head. Part the hair in the center from crown to nape. Comb down a diagonal section of hair on each side of the part. Cut off a 1-inch-wide section of hair in the center of the neck, using the back of the hand to hold the hair down.

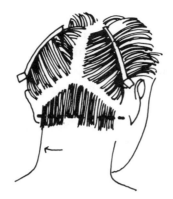

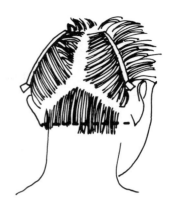

STEP 10

This will set the bottom line. When cut, the bottom line of the hair should be even with the base of the ear. Cut from center to left, then center to right until all the hair in that section is the same length.

11. Cut the pieces of hair directly behind the ears on each side to conform to the same angle as the hair over the ears. To do this, pull the hair from behind the ear forward to meet the piece covering the ear and cut to the same length and angle. As you continue bringing down sections in back, cut the hair on each side this way.

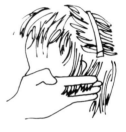

STEP 11

12. Comb down another diagonal section of hair. Starting in the center, comb up a 1-inch-thick horizontal section of hair together with a partial piece from the first layer. Hold diagonally out from the head and cut 1 inch long. Work your way from center to left, then center to right, combing new sections together with pieces from the layer underneath and cut to the same length. Make sure to angle the hair directly behind the ears.

13. Continue combing down diagonal sections of hair and cutting the top layer to match the hair underneath all the way up to the crown.

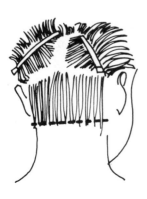

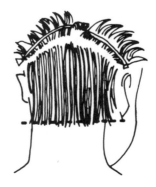

STEP 13

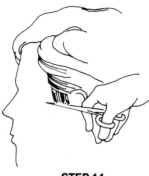

STEP 14

14. Trim sideburns. Usually the center of the ear is the right length for men's sideburns. But use your eye to judge the length that looks best. You might want to make them a little longer or shorter so they're in proportion to the length of your neck.

To start, comb the hair on the sides of the head behind the ears so the sideburns are exposed. Comb the sideburns straight down. Beginning on either side, cut the sideburn to the desired length, working from back to front. Do the same thing on the other side. Check to make sure the sideburns are even by lining up your thumbnails on either side of the head.

15. Contour the hair around the ears. The object is to cut away the hair covering the ears following the natural contour of the ears. First, comb the hair down over the ears. Beginning in front of one ear, cut the hair as closely as possible over and around the ear, taking tiny snips. Continue cutting this way until you reach the bottom of the ear in back. You may have to repeat this process several times until you've trimmed the hair in a neat line around the ear. Then repeat the same steps on the other side.

STEP 15

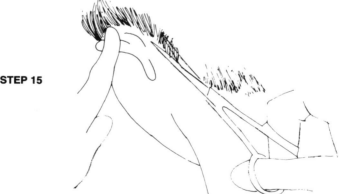

16. Clip the hair at the nape. There will be some stubbly hair left over at the nape below the bottom line. You can either shave it off or clip it off with scissors. To cut it off, hold the scissors perpendicular to the head, like a pair of clippers, and shear off the excess hair as close to the back of the neck as possible Make sure to clip the hair in the direction in which it grows. If you don't, ingrown hairs could result.

STEP 16

MODIFIED MILITARY CUT

We've modified the traditional crew cut to make it look modern. Our version is layered close to the head but not clean-shaven. As a result, it doesn't have that severe, razored look. In addition, it's a little longer on the top, which gives it volume and a definite style. It's a great warm-weather cut. And it works on all hair textures, from straight to very curly and wiry.

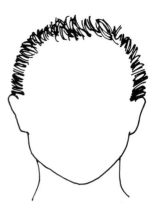

Technique: The key to this cut is a lifting motion. You'll need to master picking up a small section of uncut hair with your comb, along with a piece you've already cut from the layer beneath, lifting and cutting to the length of the short piece.

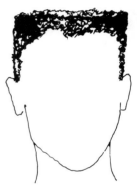

INSTRUCTIONS

1. Wash and towel dry the hair. Part it down the center in back from crown to nape and separate a diagonal wedge 1 inch above the hairline. Cut a 1-inch-wide piece in the center back to serve as your bottom line. The length should be even with the bottom of the ear. Then, using the 1-inch strip as a guide, cut to the left, then the right, holding the hair down with the back of the hand. After you've established the length of the hair in back, you're going to cut the rest very close to the scalp—1/2 to 1/4 inch in length, depending upon how short you want it.

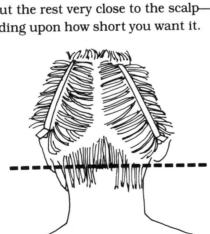

STEP 1

2. Comb down another diagonal wedge. Comb together a ½-inch-thick piece of hair from the center of the wedge you just brought down along with some hair from underneath. Now lift the hair up and cut the top layer of hair to the length of the short piece underneath. Continue lifting and cutting ½-inch pieces until you've finished the entire diagonal section.

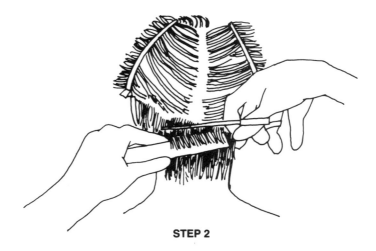

STEP 2

3. Continue combing down diagonal sections of hair and cutting them using the "lifting" technique. Your last diagonal wedge should be about 2 inches above the ear. Stop when you reach this point.

4. Now go on to the sides of the head. It doesn't matter which side you do first. Part off a horizontal section of hair 1 inch above the ear. Comb together a piece of hair from over the ear, together

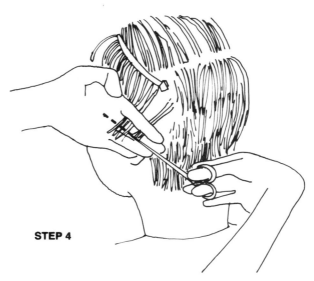

STEP 4

with a piece from the back of the head. Cut the hair over the ear to the same length as the piece in back.

5. Divide the hair in the large horizontal section into smaller pieces and cut to the same length as the guide piece you set in step 4. To do, pick up a ¹/₂-inch-thick section of hair from over the ear, together with a piece from the back, lift upward with the comb and cut to desired length. Continue dividing the hair into ¹/₂-inch sections and cut it to match the preceding piece. Work from the back of the ear forward toward the cheek.

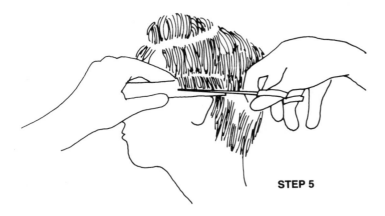

STEP 5

6. Continue combing down 1-inch-thick horizontal sections, dividing them into ¹/₂-inch pieces, lifting a little hair from the layer beneath and cutting to match the length of the shortest piece.

7. Repeat steps 4 through 6 on the other side of the head.

8. Now go on to the front of the head. Comb down a section of hair 1 inch thick from temple to temple. Starting in the center of the forehead, hold a ¹/₂-inch-thick lock of hair straight up and make a cut 1 inch wide.

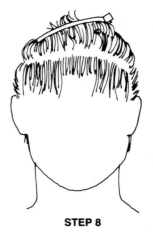

STEP 8

9. Pick up a section of hair to the left of the one you just cut. Hold it straight up, along with a piece from the center of the forehead as a guideline, and cut to the same length. Continue across the left side. Now cut the hair on the right side of the forehead to the same length as the center piece.

10. Comb down another 1-inch-thick section of hair from the front of the head. Again, starting in the middle, comb up a ¹/₂-inch-thick piece of hair from the new layer together with a piece from the layer underneath, lift up and cut to the same length as the short piece. Lift and cut all the hair in the horizontal section piece by piece, working your way from center to left, then center to right.

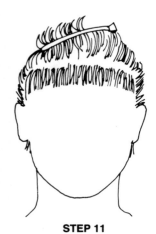

STEP 11

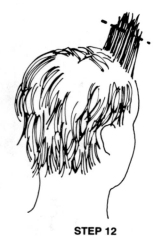

STEP 12

11. Keep bringing down horizontal sections, combing them together with pieces of hair underneath and cutting to the same length until you run out of hair that hasn't been cut.

12. The last step is to make sure there are no stray strands of long hair that you've missed on the top of the head. The back and sides are so short that they don't require checking. Here's how to do the check:

Starting from the front of the head, comb a section of hair back from the middle and hold it straight up and taut between your fingers. The hair should be even in length. If it looks longer in the center than on the sides, cut off the long piece to match the shorter pieces. Work your way back to the crown, checking sections of hair in the center of the head.

Comb the hair back diagonally over the left temple. Pick up a section closest to the hairline and see if it's longer in the middle. If it is, cut from short point to short point. Continue combing back sections of hair to check if they're even until you reach the crown. Now follow the same procedure on the right side.

Styling tip: Brush the hair backward to give it more volume. If your hair doesn't grow back naturally, use a little gel to keep it in place.

FRINGE BENEFITS—HOW TO CARE FOR A MUSTACHE AND BEARD

Whether or not to sprout whiskers is mostly a matter of personal preference. When making the decision, keep in mind that a beard or mustache probably won't make a dramatic difference in your appearance. However, they can add character to a face and make you look a bit more distinguished. If you don't already have a mustache or beard, let your hair grow for four to six weeks before you begin shaping it. Don't be surprised if your facial hair isn't the same color as the hair on your head. You may have brown hair, but a reddish mustache or beard. Or your hair may grow in partially gray. Some men even have multicolored beards—a combination of dark brown, light brown and gray hair, for instance.

Mustaches

The most common type of mustache is a simple cropped type that fills out the area from the base of the nose to the edge of the upper lip and extends out to the corners of the mouth. If your upper lip is very thin, however, you might want to let your mustache grow over the edge of the lip slightly to camouflage it. On the other hand, if your mouth is nicely shaped, trim your mustache above your upper lip to show it off.

TRIMMING A MUSTACHE

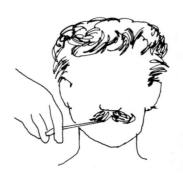

Shaping a mustache couldn't be simpler. To start, comb hair straight down. If it curves to one side, cut it in the direction it grows in. Don't try to force the hair to lie down straight.

Hold the scissors on a diagonal at the corner of the mouth. Now make small snips right above the edge of the upper lip all the way across to the opposite corner.

Beards

The classic beard connects with the sideburns and mustache and grows under the chin. There are two basic beard shapes: round and square. A round beard is cut to conform to the shape of the face. It's best for very curly hair and will camouflage a protruding jaw. A square beard is cut on an angle at the jawline, and works best on straight hair. The square beard can also make a receding chin look more prominent.

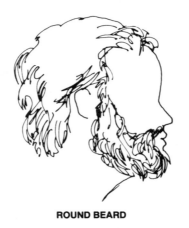

ROUND BEARD

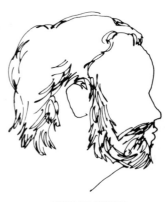

SQUARE BEARD

A note on length: You're going to have to be the judge of how long or short to make your beard, but a moderate look is best. The density of facial hair is purely individual. In general, your beard should be in proportion with the hair on your head. If your hair has a lot of volume, or if you wear it on the longish side, you can wear a longer, fuller beard. If your hair is short or sparse, though, you should clip your beard close to the face. Your stature and body type play a role in how much facial hair you can flaunt, too. A tall man with a big build can carry off a bushy beard far better than a man who is slight.

TRIMMING A BEARD

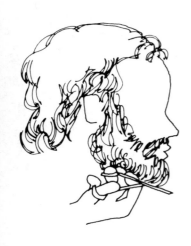

Technique: There's a method to trimming a beard. It's called "free-handing." Holding the scissors parallel to the face, and using them like a pair of clippers, trim the hair all over the face, taking small snips.

Trimming   Comb the hair upward and outward. Whether you're shaping a round or square beard, trim the hair on one side of the face, then the other. Start at the center of the chin, holding the scissors parallel to the face. For a round beard, trim the hair to the desired length in small snips, following the contours of the face. Work your way outward and upward to the cheek. Then go back to the center of the chin and trim the hair on the other side the same way.

For a square shape, cut the bottom of the beard on one side of the face in a straight line. Then work your way over to the jawline, trimming the hair to the length you've decided upon. Cut the hair along the jawline at a right angle. Continue cutting the hair outward and upward. When you reach the cheek, taper the hair closer to the face. Follow the same steps on the other side of the face.

Tip: If your beard is partly gray or more than one shade, make sure to cut the lighter hair the same length as the dark areas. The light sections may appear shorter than the dark areas, so the tendency is to make them a little too long. As a result, your beard may come out uneven.

GROOMING A BEARD

A beard requires the same kind of care as the hair on your head. Shampoo it when you wash your hair. To keep it looking neat, first comb it out from the face. Then smooth down the outer layer with the comb to emphasize the shape of the beard. Dab on a little cologne to keep it fresh.

HOW TO HIDE OR DISGUISE THAT BALD OR THIN SPOT

Losing your hair can be traumatic. But there's not much you can do to prevent hair loss—it's hereditary. (Using a protein conditioner after shampooing, however, will help make your hair stronger.) Progressive hair loss, called "male pattern alopecia," occurs along the hairline in front of the head on the crown. It's normal to lose between 50 and 100 hairs per day. If hair loss is heavy or starts in the late teens or early twenties, it's usually a sign that you're going bald.

There are better ways to camouflage a balding pate than by plastering hair across your forehead, letting the fringe below a bald spot grow long and straggly or wearing a phony-looking hairpiece. Following are some of the most common problems that accompany hair loss and the clever cutting techniques that will disguise them. They're all based upon the first style in this section, the short layered men's cut.

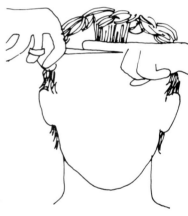

Problem: Thinning or bald pate surrounded by a fringe of hair.

Solution: Cut hair in short, even layers, no longer than 1 inch. Keeping your hair short and neatly trimmed will create the illusion of more hair. Curly hair, because it expands, will look especially thick when cut this way.

Problem: Receding hairline at the temples.

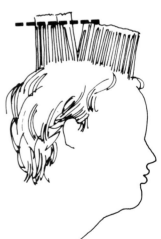

Solution: The trick here is to layer the hair so it falls over the forehead and disguises the recession at the temples. When following the men's layered cut, cut the first piece of hair in front of the head over the forehead 1 inch long. It will be your guideline for layering the hair in the front of the head.

If the hair over the temple is sparse, pull down the piece of hair directly behind it and cut to the same length as the piece over the forehead. When you reach the crown, match the last section of hair from the front of the head to the last section that you did in the back to blend in the layers.

Problem: A bald or thinning spot at the top or back of the head.

Solution: Match the length of the layer in front of the bald spot with the layer behind it. If you come across an area that's thinning and has short pieces, don't cut them. Just skip over that spot and match the sections on each side.

Haircutting and Styling for Children and Teens

Children's hair requires special care. In this section, we've included information for kids of all ages—tender treatment for newborns, easy-care cuts for toddlers and new twists for teens. When kids reach kindergarten age, you can give them any one of the haircuts for adults in this book. The styling tricks will tell teenage girls how to get a great new look by braiding, twisting and tying their hair in different ways.

TAKING CARE OF BABY

Whether your baby is born with a layer of downy peach fuzz or a headful of hair, treat your baby's hair with tender loving care. It's fragile and the skin on your baby's scalp is delicate. At birth, a baby's skull isn't fully formed. There's a soft spot at the crown where the bones of the skull haven't yet grown together. New mothers may be afraid to wash an infant's hair for fear of injuring the tender spot. To keep a baby's hair clean and healthy, however, frequent shampooing is a must. Newborns are vulnerable to cradle cap, a condition that causes a flaky, oily coating on the crown of a child's head. No one is sure exactly what causes it, but lack of shampooing could be a contributing factor. If your baby does get cradle cap, consult a pediatrician who can prescribe the correct treatment. Following are the how-tos of caring for your baby's hair. When your child is big enough to take a regular bath, wash his or her hair the way you do your own.

INSTRUCTIONS

1. Shampooing should be done at baby's bath time. Fill a little inflatable tub with lukewarm water.
2. Pour a little baby shampoo into a dish and place it within

arm's reach of the tub. Wet the baby's head by cupping handfuls of water in your hand, from the tub.

3. Dab your fingers into the baby shampoo and, using the pads of your fingertips, gently swab the baby's entire head. Scoop up handfuls of water from the tub to rinse the baby's hair. Pat the scalp dry with a soft towel.

NO-FUSS CUTS FOR TODDLERS

TIPS ON TAMING A TODDLER DURING A HAIRCUT

Most children, unless they're born with a bountiful head of hair, need their first haircut when they're about a year old. Here are some pointers on how to get great results when cutting the hair of a small child.

- Getting a youngster to sit still for any length of time is no easy task. A story or a game during haircutting can keep the kids occupied. For instance, you could tell the child that every time he or she moves when you snip off a piece of hair, you get a point. The child gets a point for staying still during each snip of the scissors. (The odds of course are heavily stacked in the haircutter's favor.)
- Use a pair of scissors with blunt tips to avoid mishaps with a child.
- Make sure the child is sitting up straight in the chair; otherwise the hair may come out uneven.
- Children who are getting their first haircut may become anxious because they're afraid it will hurt. Reassure the child that the process is painless. You might even demonstrate by snipping a small piece of your own hair.

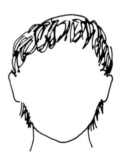

THE QUICK ONE-STEP CUT

This cut is perfect for active youngsters. It's a simplified version of the layered cut, so it's quick and easy to do. It isn't necessary to part off and clip up the hair in this style, so you can get your little one in and out of the barber's chair in a jiffy.

The technique involves cutting from front hairline to the neckline in three sections: down the center of the head and diagonally on each side. When you're finished, you get a soft, tousled look that frames the face. You can part the hair on the side or comb it forward onto the face—whichever way it looks best. The cut is

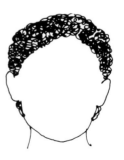

cute on both boys and girls. And it's perfect for all textures of hair—straight, wavy, curly and wiry.

INSTRUCTIONS

1. Wash and towel dry the hair. Comb it straight back off the face.

2. Begin in front. Comb down a ½-inch-thick section of hair 1 inch back from the hairline in the center of the forehead. Hold the hair straight up with the comb and cut off 1 to 2 inches.

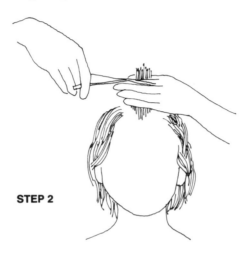

STEP 2

3. Comb up another section directly in back of the first. Blend in a little bit of the hair from the first section you cut and snip the hair to match the short piece.

4. Continue cutting consecutive sections of hair using the preceding piece as a guideline, all the way back to the nape of the neck.

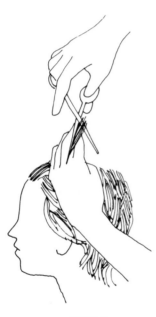

STEP 3

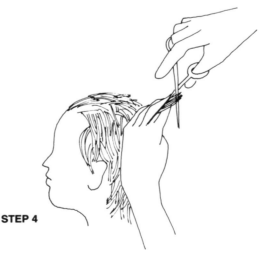

STEP 4

5. Now return to the front of the head. You're going to cut the hair on one side in a triangular section. The widest point of the triangle stretches from the tip of the eyebrow to the top of the ear. The narrowest point is at the crown.

Separate a ½-inch section of hair 1 inch back from the hairline over the corner of the brow. Comb it straight up, blending in a little hair from the first cut you made in the center of the forehead. Hold the hair taut out from the head at the angle in which the hair grows. Then cut the hair to match the short piece.

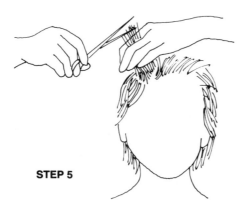

STEP 5

6. Comb up another diagonal section. Blend in some hair from the section in front of it that you just cut and snip to equal length. Work your way back to the crown, parting off diagonal sections and cutting them to the length of the piece in front of them. You'll notice that the triangular section of hair you started out with will begin narrowing as you work your way toward the crown.

7. Repeat the same steps on the other side of the head, first pulling up a section of hair 1 inch back from the hairline over the corner of the brow. Cut it to match the piece you snipped from the center. Then continue combing up diagonal sections and cutting them to the length of the pieces preceding them until you reach the crown.

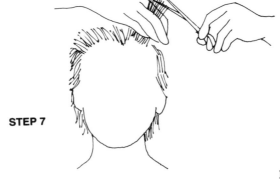

STEP 7

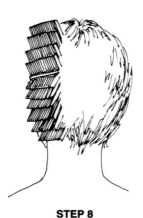

STEP 8

8. Next, cut the hair on the sides in back to match the center strip you already cut from front to nape. Starting behind one ear, comb a section of hair out from the head on the diagonal, along with a piece from the crown that you already cut. Hold the hair taut and cut to the length of the short piece. Pick up another section of hair, together with a piece from above it, and snip to equal length. Work your way down to the nape combing the sections straight out from the head and matching them to the preceding sections.

9. Now repeat step 8 on the other side, again beginning behind the ear.

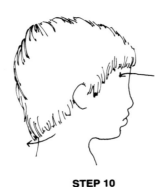

STEP 10

10. Comb the front and sides forward and the rest of the hair into shape. Now you'll trim the edges all around the head to clean up the line. Trim the edges in front first, pressing the hair down against the head with the flat of your hand. Cut the hair in an even line, taking small snips. Work your way down one side. Then do the other.

11. Last, do the back. Take off excess length by cutting the hair to mid-neck level or a little longer.

To style the hair, you can part it in the center or on the side or comb it forward onto the face.

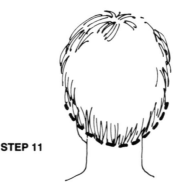

STEP 11

THE BOWL CUT

Here's a classic cut for little boys and girls that takes a few more steps than the previous one. The hair is lightly layered so it falls into a soft, smooth shape. What makes this cut unique is the curved shape. You achieve it by cutting the hair in an inverted U shape around the face. This style is for straight hair, from fine to thick-textured. Curly hair won't conform to the line of the bowl cut.

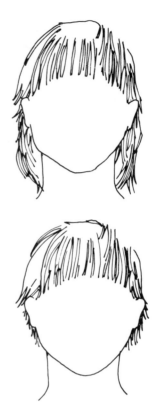

Before cutting the hair in an inverted U shape, visualize the line you're going to create. Again, it's helpful to use facial features such as the brows and cheekbones as markers for where to cut the hair.

INSTRUCTIONS

1. Wash and towel dry the hair. Part it down the center in back and comb down a diagonal wedge 1 inch above the hairline. Clip the rest of the hair up and out of the way. Measure down three to four thumb lengths from the base of the skull—this is where to set your bottom line. Holding down the hair with the back of your hand, cut off a 1-inch-wide section in the center. Then cut from this notch out to each side, using small snips.

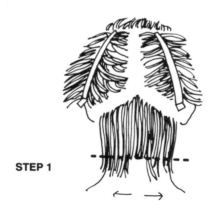

STEP 1

2. Part off another diagonal wedge of hair 1 inch higher than the last one and comb it over the section you just finished. At this point, you're going to begin layering the hair vertically.

Comb up a ½-inch-thick piece of hair from the center of the head, together with a piece of hair from the section underneath. Hold the hair straight out from the head and cut to the length of the short bottom layer. Working from center to left, continue dividing the hair into vertical pieces containing hair from the

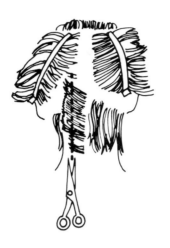 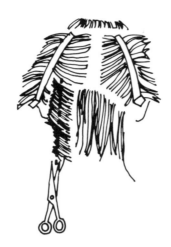

layer underneath and cutting it to the length of the short piece. Then continue to cut the hair in vertical pieces from center to right.

3. Proceed up the head, parting off horizontal sections of hair 1 inch apart, dividing them into vertical pieces and cutting them to equal length.

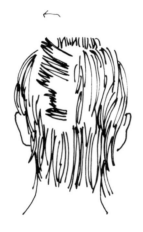 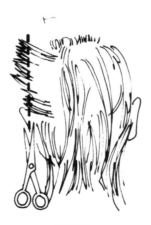 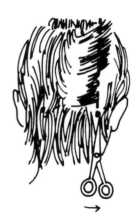

STEP 3

4. When you reach the crown, part the hair from ear to ear. Comb down a 1-inch-thick horizontal section over one ear. Clip the hair above it up and out of the way. Pull a piece of hair from in back forward to meet the hair over the ear. Comb the pieces together, hold taut between index and middle finger and cut to the length of the short piece from the back. Comb down a horizontal section on the other side of the head and cut the same way.

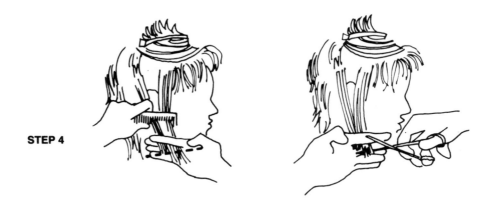

STEP 4

5. Now go around to the front of the head. Part the hair down the center. Bring down a 1-inch section of hair from part to back of ear on the left side. Comb the hair straight down over the forehead and on the sides of the head. Now holding the piece of hair over the forehead taut, cut it off right below the brow. Continue cutting the hair around the face in an inverted U shape from the temple to the center of the earlobe. The hair should curve around the tip of the eyebrow and the top of the cheekbone and slope gently around the ear. If you like, you can use a water-soluble marking pen to draw the pattern on the face to use as your guide when cutting. Do not press the hair against the head when creating the shape of this cut—you may distort the line.

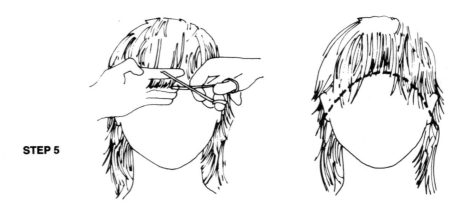

STEP 5

6. Cut the hair on the other side of the head exactly the same way. Separate a 1-inch section of hair from part to ear and comb it straight down. Begin by matching up the hair on the right side of the forehead with the piece you already cut on the left side. Then cut the hair in an inverted U shape, conforming to the same line you created on the other side.

7. Go back to the left side and separate another 1-inch section of hair from part to ear. Now you're going to layer the hair vertically, the way you did in back. Begin next to the part and comb a ½-inch-thick section of hair straight up, together with a piece of hair from the layer over the forehead. Cut to the length of the short piece from the front. Separate another section right beneath the one you just cut. Mix in a little hair from the first layer you cut and snip to equal length. Work your way down the head to the ear, cutting the hair vertically. Hold the hair out diagonally as you proceed toward the bottom of the ear. Repeat this step on the right side.

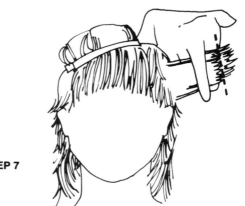

STEP 7

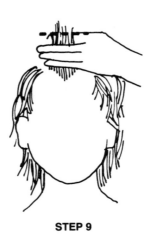

8. Continue alternating from left to right, separating ½-inch-thick vertical layers of hair from part to ear on each side of the head, until you run out of hair. When you're done, the hair will softly frame the face.

9. Check to see if you've layered the hair evenly. Start at the center of the forehead and comb a 1-inch-thick section of hair straight up. If a long piece of hair is sticking out, cut it off. Work your way across the head and down the nape, checking for long pieces. Comb horizontal sections of hair up diagonally over the left temple and check for long pieces, working your way down to the nape. Comb up diagonal sections from right temple to nape and check for long pieces that you've missed.

STEP 9

HAIR REPAIR CUT

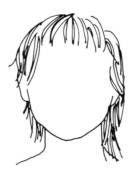

The most common type of hair emergency is when a long-haired little girl gives herself a "haircut" by chopping off a chunk of her hair. Don't despair. Repairing the hair might not be as hard as you think. The cut uses vertical layers in a circular pattern to camouflage the gaps.

The first thing to do is assess the damage. If she's cut off a patch of hair on the top or side of the head, you may be able to camouflage it by combing the hair closest to the face over it. For instance, pulling the hair back into pigtails, a ponytail or a braid, will disguise the spot. If the hair is short on the side, try gathering a section of hair into a butterfly clip or barrette and fastening it over the shorn area.

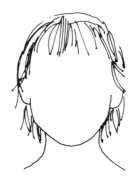

If the hair is much shorter on one side and cut in choppy layers on the other, you may have to take more drastic measures. To repair the hair, you'll have to layer it, following the directions below. If the hair is cut off very close to the scalp, however, it's best to let a professional handle the problem. The lopped-off hair should be at least a few inches long to do our cut.

INSTRUCTIONS

1. Shampoo hair and towel dry. Part the hair on the side or in the center, where you usually do.

2. Even out the length of the hair on the side where the accident happened by cutting off rough edges or long pieces from the bottom.

3. Cut the hair in back to the same length as the hair over the ear. Judge how many inches you have to cut off in back so the bottom will be even with the short side. You can use your thumb as a ruler. From the tip of the thumb down to the first joint is about 1 inch.

The next five steps are exactly the same as for the blunt cut in "Haircutting and Styling for Women." So you don't have to flip back and forth through the book, we've included them here, again.

4. Part the hair down the center from crown to nape. Part off two diagonal sections of hair 1 inch above the hairline on each side. Comb them straight down against the nape. Clip the rest of the hair out of the way. Starting in the center of the head, cut off

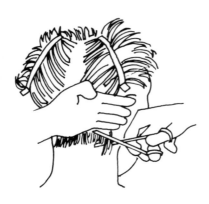
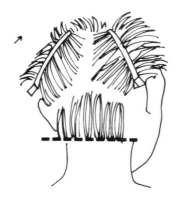

STEP 4

a 1-inch-wide section to use as your guideline. Hold the hair down with the back of your hand so it lies flat. Then continue cutting the same length from center to left and center to right.

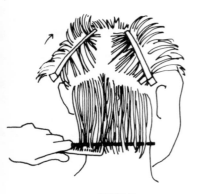

STEP 5

5. Comb down two more diagonal pieces of hair 1 inch above the original ones. Using the bottom layer of hair as your guideline, continue cutting the hair the same length from the center out to the sides.

6. Work your way up to the crown, combing down diagonal sections of hair 1 inch apart. Cut them to the same length as the hair underneath.

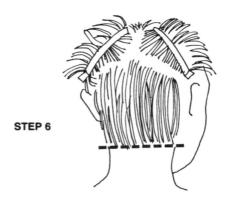

STEP 6

7. Go on to the side of the hair your child didn't cut. Part the hair from ear to ear all the way across the crown. Comb down a horizontal section 1 inch above the ear. Pull forward a piece of hair from behind the ear and comb together with the piece over the ear. Hold taut between your fingers as close to the face as possible and cut to the length of the short piece from the back.

8. Continue combing down horizontal sections of hair and cutting them to the same length as the sections underneath them until you reach the part.

9. Now you're going to layer the hair. Look for the shortest piece among the choppy layers your child cut. You're going to cut the rest of the hair the same length.

Comb the shortest piece up vertically from the head, together with a 1-inch-thick piece of hair from below it. Hold the hair straight out from the head and cut to the length of the short piece.

10. Continue cutting the hair below the shortest piece. Then cut the hair above it in vertical sections up to the part until you've layered one whole side of the hair.

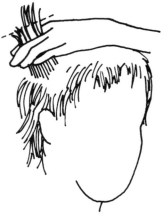

STEP 9

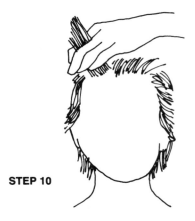

STEP 10

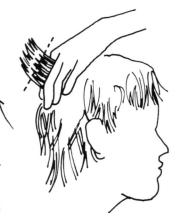

STEP 11

11. Go on to the back of the head. Comb together a piece of hair from the top of the head with a vertical section of hair from behind the ear. Hold the hair straight out from the head and cut to the length of the short piece. *Tip:* Take large vertical sections that stretch from crown to the base of skull. You'll be able to do this because a child's head is so small. If some hair falls out of your hand, let it go and cut it in a separate vertical section along with the piece above it as your guide.

12. Comb up another vertical section from crown to base of the neck. Mix in a little hair from the section behind the ear and cut to the length of the short piece.

13. Move across the head to the opposite ear, dividing the hair into large vertical sections and cutting them to the length of the previous sections.

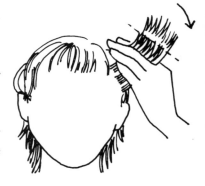

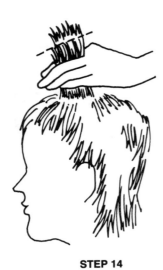

STEP 14

14. Layer the hair on the opposite side of the part. Comb up a vertical section of hair together with a piece from the top of the head on the top of the head on the other side. Cut to the length of the short piece.

15. Comb up a vertical section of hair beneath the one you just cut. Mix in a piece of already cut hair and snip to the same length. Work your way down to the ear, cutting the hair in vertical sections containing a piece from the previous layer.

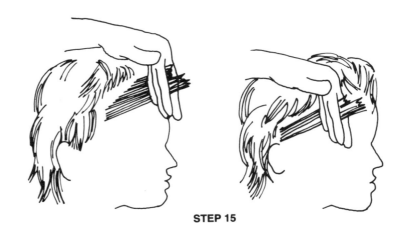

STEP 15

HAIR CARE FOR TEENS

Due to hormonal changes that take place in the body during puberty, the sebaceous, or, oil glands produce excess oil. The oil is usually associated with bad skin—breakouts and acne. But it can also affect the hair and make it excessively greasy. The scalp is, after all, skin. Oily hair can develop an unpleasant odor caused by a combination of dirt, oils and perspiration. Teens may also be especially prone to dandruff.

Oily, stringy hair and broken-out skin can make any teenager unhappy and self-conscious. That's why teens must take extra care to keep their hair and skin sparkling clean. But some kids may go overboard. Rough treatment of the skin and scalp and harsh shampoos and soaps should be avoided. Dryness and irritation may result.

To control oiliness and keep hair fresh, you should wash it frequently; twice a day if necessary, with a shampoo formulated for oily hair. If you notice flaking, use a dandruff shampoo to cleanse the scalp. In a pinch, when there's no time to shampoo, such as after gym class, try dabbing the scalp with witch hazel applied with a cotton ball. It will absorb some of the oil on the scalp.

FOR GIRLS ONLY—STYLING TIPS

You don't have to cut or perm your hair to get a whole new look. Next time you want a change of pace, try some of the following tricks. They'll jazz up your everyday style or add glamour for night. They're easy and inexpensive to do.

BRIGHTENING TRICKS

Fizz-In-Highlights   To bring out the natural radiance in your hair, spray on a colored mousse. You'll find a variety of flavors. There's lemon for blonds, strawberry for redheads and chocolate for brunettes. The color is temporary and washes out with your next shampoo.

Chamomile Brightener   To give blond hair a lift, pick up some chamomile tea at a health food store. Brew a pot of tea using two tea bags. Let steep. When completely cool, rinse the tea through your hair.

Apple Cider Rinse   To get any shade of hair its shiniest, add ½ cup of cider vinegar to 2 cups of water and pour through your hair. The vinegar restores the pH balance to the hair and makes it look lustrous. It also removes any shampoo, which can dull the hair.

BODY BUILDER

Quick Lift   Here's a great way to add fullness to your hair. Blow it dry until just damp, then apply a little mousse or gel to your fingers. Starting anywhere, slip your fingers through your hair, close to the scalp. Then lift the roots of your hair lightly. Continue lifting your hair all over your head, until it has the height you want. If you like, blow-dry your hair as you lift it so it looks fluffier.

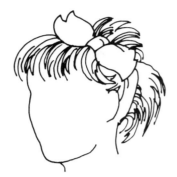

PRETTY ACCESSORIES

Ritzy Rags If you want to dress up your hair instantly, here's a trick modeled after Madonna's hairstyle. All you need is a strip of gauze or cotton fabric. Or you can cut a strip of fabric from an old T-shirt. This look works on any length of hair but looks especially pretty if you have a bob. Tie the fabric around your head candy-box style, off to one side, and make a bow or knot in it. Then, using your fingers, fluff your hair out around it. For night, try tying on a ribbon in satin, moire, taffeta or eyelet.

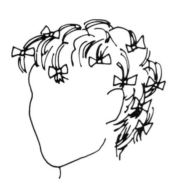

Tiny Ties If you're the adventurous type, you might want to try this idea. It looks great even on short hair. To do, tie bows at the end of thin sections of hair, randomly over your head or just on each side. You can even tie bows in your bangs.

Butterfly Clips These overgrown clips make terrific hair ornaments. Use them like barrettes or combs to pull your hair back off your face. Use more than one for dazzling designs. Here's a pattern you can make using three small to medium-sized clips. Pull all the hair on one side back with a clip. Then just for decoration, put in another clip so it lines up evenly with the first one. Add another clip so you have three ornaments in a row.

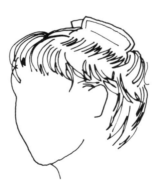 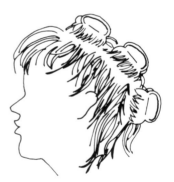

SIMPLE SETS

Piping Up For a wavy effect, try setting hair on pipe cleaners. This set works on hair that's all one length or layered. Begin by dampening your hair, then work in a little mousse or gel for more holding power. Bend the pipe cleaner in half to form a U. Starting

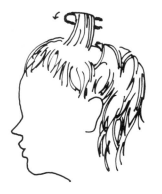 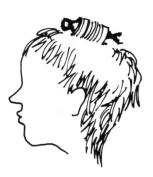

anywhere, roll up a ½-inch-thick section of hair over and around the U of the pipe cleaner, then twist the ends together to close. Roll up same-size sections of hair all over your head until all of it is set. When dry, brush out your hair lightly. If your hair is straight, you might want to set only your bangs on pipe cleaners for an interesting contrast in textures.

Bag It   If your hair is all one length and comes down to your chin or below, here's how to get a headful of gentle curls. Cut a stiff brown paper bag into long inch-wide strips. You're going to use the strips as curlers. Dampen hair and work some mousse or gel through it. Starting anywhere, separate a ½-inch-thick section of hair. Hold the paper strip out on a right angle from the section of hair you've separated and place the ends of the hair on top of the strip. Now begin rolling the hair over the strip all the way to the scalp. Then tie the ends in a knot to hold it in place. Section the hair all over the head and roll it up in separate strips. When your hair is dry, take it down, and, for maximum volume, simply ruffle up your curls with your fingers. If you'd prefer a softer, fuller look, lightly brush your hair.

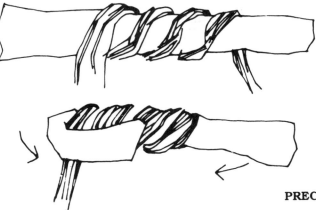

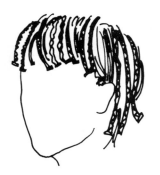

Make Waves Dampen hair and braid it in ½-inch-thick sections all over the head. Use small metal hair clips to secure the braids—they're much easier to handle and kinder to the hair than rubber bands. Let hair air-dry. Then comb out with your fingers so your hair falls in fluffy waves. For a crimped look, set hair in smaller braids.

BEAUTIFUL BRAIDS

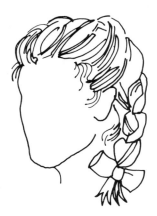

Side Sweep For a romantic style that's perfect for a party, braid all your hair loosely to one side. Then tie a satin bow in a pastel color at the end of the braid. Pull a few wisps of hair down at the front and sides of your head to frame your face.

Woven Wonder This is a jazzed-up version of the standard braid. Pull your hair back and separate into three even pieces. Before you actually start braiding, tie a long, thin strip of ribbon to the top of each section of hair. Make the knots underneath so they won't show. Now weave the ribbons into your hair as you braid it. Try using two or three different colors of ribbon for a special effect.

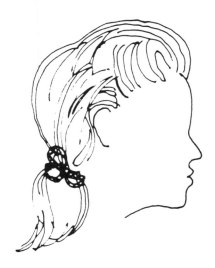

Fabulous Fakes If you have medium to long hair, you can create some great styles with artificial braids. Pick up half a dozen braids 12 to 12½ inches long and about ¼ inch wide from a wig store. Choose braids that are the same shade as your hair or get a mixture of complementary colors. If you have blond hair, weave in light brown and strawberry blond braids. For light brown or red hair, mix in brown and blond braids. On brunette hair use silver and reddish braids. Here are some looks you might want to try:

• Put your hair in a regular ponytail and secure it with a coated elastic band. Then tie a braid in a bow around it so it looks like a hair ornament.

• For a glamorous nighttime look, put your hair up into a chignon, then wrap braids around it so it looks like a jewel in a beautiful setting. To do, put your hair in a ponytail at the crown or the nape of the neck, depending on where you want the chignon. You could also make ponytails on each side of the head for two small chignons. Wind the hair around the base of the ponytail to form a bun. Slip some small hairpins (the same color as your hair) under the edges of the chignon. For a more sophisticated look, you can twist the tail into a coil before wrapping it into a chignon. To keep the chignon in place, pin an invisible hair net over it that matches. Now decorate the chignon with braids.

Take four braids together and twist them into a single rope. Then wrap them around the base of the chignon and pin underneath with hairpins.

Another idea: Take six braids together so they're parallel to each other, then tie them in a bow. Pin the bow on top of the chignon.

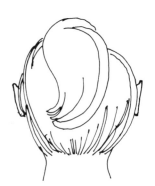 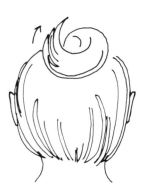 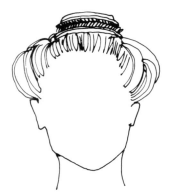

A NEW TWIST

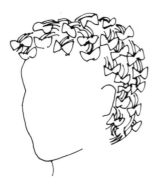

Springy Curls This style is great for medium to long hair that's wiry and very curly. Divide your hair into large sections in the front, back and sides. Comb gel into the front, then brush until smooth. Now divide the hair in the large section into smaller pieces. Take a ½-inch-thick section of hair and twist it tightly from roots to ends to form curlicues. Repeat, working in gel on the sides. Then do the back of your hair. If you like, tie the twists with a piece of fabric.

SPECIAL EFFECTS 4

Perfect Perms

A perm gives you a wonderful kind of freedom. It lets you have the texture of hair you wish you'd been born with. A perm can add body and fullness to your hair or create waves or curls. Your hair will be easy to care for too, because you can simply wash it, ruffle it up with your fingers and go. There's no need for time-consuming setting or styling.

First decide on what kind of look you want. A variety of formulas are available that will produce natural-looking effects. The package label will tell you the result you can expect. A "body wave" will make your hair look thicker and more voluminous. It's an especially good choice if your hair is fine or if it won't hold a set. With this type of perm your hair will have more bounce and maintain its shape better. A body wave works well on blunt-cut or layered hair.

Other types of perms will create a marked change in your hair texture. If you'd like soft waves or curls, choose a perm marked "regular" on the package. For lots of tight curls, get an "extra curly" perm. A wavy or curly perm is best for layered hair. Layering will play up your new curls and make the hair look fuller and fluffier. If your hair is all one length, however, waves or curls will droop.

Another factor to take into consideration when choosing a perm is your hair texture. Perms are made for normal and hard-to-curl hair (which can be fine or coarse) and color-treated hair. Select the formula that suits your hair type.

Home perms now on the market are formulated to be gentle to the hair and simple to use. All perms, however, contain strong chemicals and must be used with care. A perm changes the structure of the hair and gives it a new shape. It's a two-step process. First you apply a waving solution to weaken the chemical bonds that give the hair its natural texture. The hair will then conform to the shape of the permanent rods (curlers) it's set on. The tightness of the curl depends upon the size of the rods you use. The larger they are the softer the curl will be (see the "Perm Checklist" below for more details). You leave on the waving solution for the time specified in the directions, then rinse it out. During the second step, you saturate the hair with a "neutralizer" which locks the hair into its new shape. The neutralizer is not a conditioner. Don't leave it on any longer than directed.

There are times when it's not advisable to perm the hair. If it's dry, brittle or damaged, perming it will only aggravate the problem. Perming your hair when your scalp is sensitive, irritated or cut could be harmful to your health. Don't do it.

PERM CHECKLIST

The permanent kit you buy will provide the waving solution and a plastic cap to cover your head after applying it, neutralizer and endpapers to protect the ends of the hair. Deluxe kits come with rods to set the hair on, but basic kits do not; you'll have to buy them at a beauty supply store. Perm rods come in different colors, depending upon the size of the curl they create. Pink or gray rods are the smallest and produce the tightest curls. Purple rods create soft curls; beige rods result in loose waves. White rods create the loosest wave. The instructions in the perm kit will tell you what size rod to get. In addition to the contents of the kit, you'll need the following items:

A *plastic rat-tail comb* to separate sections of hair before you roll them on the rods. Do not use a metal comb; the chemicals in the perm will react badly with the metal.

A *roll of cotton* that comes in a long, thin strand to wrap around the head after applying the waving solution.

A *spray nozzle* that attaches to your sink so you can rinse your hair thoroughly between steps.

HOME PERM TIPS

Before you begin, read the package instructions thoroughly, and follow them precisely. Keep in mind that directions do vary from brand to brand. Even if you've used a particular brand of perm previously, reread the directions before you proceed; they may have been changed or revised since the last time you used the product. Supplement the how-tos that come with the kit with the following tips. They'll help you perm your hair like a pro.

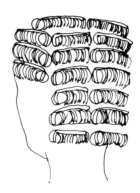

- To ensure the best results, have a friend perm your hair for you. Don't try to do it yourself. It's difficult to roll the hair quickly and accurately when you're working alone. Applying the waving solution and neutralizing lotion by yourself can also be tricky.
- Don't condition your hair before a perm. It may interfere with how well the perm penetrates the hair shaft.
- The hair should be soaking wet when it's wrapped on the perm rods. Wet hair is easier to set and will absorb the waving solution better than dry hair.
- Set the hair in equal-sized pieces all over the head. If you don't, your perm may look uneven—straight in some parts and curly in others. Here's the right way to roll up the hair: with the rat-tail comb, part off a piece of hair ¼ inch thick and 3 inches wide, or no wider than the length of the roller. Comb out the section and hold the hair straight out at a 90-degree angle from the head. Then fold the endpaper over the hair and slide it down to the bottom of the section. Very important: The ends of the hair should be completely covered. Now wind the hair under the rod. It should be smooth and flat when wrapped around the rod. Wind rollers firmly but not tightly so they rest comfortably on the head. Make sure the ends of the hair aren't bunched up inside the roller or sticking out—they might come out frizzy or hooked—a surefire sign of a poorly done home permanent.

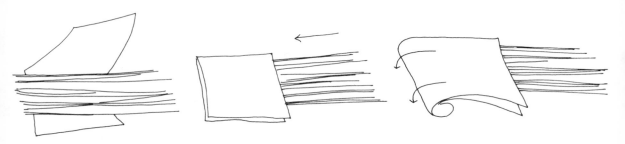

- Rinse out waving solution thoroughly with the spray nozzle. Make sure you don't disturb the rollers.
- When applying neutralizer, saturate each curl. Wait the exact amount of time specified on the package, then remove rods gently and rinse hair again. Let it air-dry.

MAINTAINING A PERM

Don't wash or condition your hair for at least 48 hours after perming it. If you do, you may take out some of the curl. A perm will be tightest right after it's done, so if your hair looks curlier than you'd like at first, don't become alarmed. Your hair will relax within a week or two.

A perm or body wave will hold two or three months. Regular trims will help make it last longer and keep curls bouncy. Apply mousse or gel before styling for extra body. If you have a body wave, you can set your hair on rollers or blow it dry on the warm setting for maximum volume. You can let a wavy or curly perm dry naturally or use a diffuser attachment to blow it dry. Scrunch your hair with your fingers as it dries to enhance the texture. Condition your hair with a protein conditioner twice a month after perming to keep it healthy.

PERM PROBLEMS

There are two things that can go wrong when you perm your hair. If you wash the waving solution out too soon, underprocessing may occur. As a result your perm may not take and your hair may look limp or stringy. When you leave the waving solution on too long, the opposite problem may happen: your hair may be overprocessed. It will look dry, frizzy and flyaway. Do not reperm your hair right away if you over- or underprocess it. You could severely damage it by applying more chemicals to freshly processed hair. Intensive conditioning is the remedy for both of these problems. Condition it once or twice a week with a protein conditioner until it returns to normal, then reperm.

PERMING COLOR-TREATED HAIR

It's safe both to color and perm your hair, but you must wait at least one week between processes. Always perm your hair first.

You can apply color over a perm, but you can't color your hair and then perm it. A perm or body wave can lift the color or change it slightly. To avoid damaging your hair, it's best to stick to a simple coloring process such as highlighting. The chemicals in hair colorings and permanents can have a doubly drying effect on your hair, so it's a good idea to step up conditioning. Use an instant conditioner after every shampoo and deep conditioner every 10 days. But try to avoid overconditioning. Perming and coloring will make the hair more porous and it may absorb too much conditioner and look limp.

Relaxing Hair

If you have very curly hair, you might want to straighten it. Relaxed hair gives you a wide variety of styling options—it can be worn any way you like. However, we don't recommend relaxing hair at home. There are several reasons why we suggest you find a professional to do the job. All relaxers contain lye, an extremely strong chemical. The amount of lye in newer formulas has been reduced, but nevertheless, a certain amount of this chemical is necessary to straighten the hair. Lye can potentially damage the hair and scalp if not applied properly. Speed is important when working with a relaxer and if you're inexperienced, you may not be able to complete the steps quickly. Also, relaxers vary greatly in quality and a professional will know which products yield the best results. A good relaxer will leave your hair shiny and smooth.

It's very important that your scalp be healthy before your hair is relaxed. Never relax the hair if the scalp is tender, sore or cut. In addition, avoid shampooing your hair for at least 24 hours before you have your hair straightened. This will help ensure that the skin on the scalp is calm and not irritated before the application. Following are the steps your hairdresser should follow when relaxing the hair:

The initial application is always done on short hair. Then you can let your hair grow as long as you like and just retouch the roots. The hair is sectioned off all over the head into ½-inch pieces with a rat-tail comb. Mineral oil is spritzed on the scalp with a misting bottle to protect it from the chemicals. Wearing gloves, the hairdresser will smooth relaxer over the top layer of the hair to begin softening it. Next, he or she will divide hair into 1-inch sections and comb relaxer through each piece from roots to ends, working from the front to the back of the head. The chemicals should be kept off the scalp and applied to the hair only. Your hairdresser will continue to comb relaxer through your hair until it reaches the desired texture. If at any time your scalp burns or begins to feel uncomfortable, ask the hairdresser to rinse out the relaxer immediately. When the hair is straight, the relaxer is rinsed out with lukewarm water. Then the hair is shampooed several times to remove all traces of chemicals and a deep conditioner is applied for 20 to 30 minutes.

You'll require touch-ups every six to seven weeks as the curly hair begins to grow in. If you wait too long between touch-ups, breakage may occur because the virgin hair will weigh down and put pressure on the fragile ends. Touch-ups are quicker than a whole-head application. Again, the scalp will be sprayed with mineral oil. Then the relaxer is applied to the new growth only. If the ends of the hair are a little frizzy, the solution can be worked through the ends of the hair for a minute or two just before it's rinsed out.

After your hair is relaxed, it can be styled any way you like by setting or blow-drying and can be worn at any length. Use a mousse or a light styling spray to give your hair more body. A sheen spray will make it look glossy.

Condition your hair once a week with a deep conditioner to keep it in good condition. If you'd like to color your hair after relaxing it, henna is your best bet (how-tos are coming up on pages 120 to 121). Do not apply hair colors containing peroxide to relaxed hair. Even a small amount of peroxide, as little as 5 percent, will cause breakage on relaxed hair.

Hair Coloring Cues

A beautiful, vibrant shade of hair can subtract years from your looks. If you'd like to perk up a dull, drab head of hair or eliminate gray, you might want to consider coloring it. The trend in hair coloring today is "less is more." A minimum of color is applied to create maximum impact.

Your natural hair color is never flat; it has a variety of tones. The new look in coloring is totally natural too—hair that shimmers with highlights. You can get great results when coloring your hair at home. The key is choosing a product that will achieve the effect you want. From simple highlights to a whole new color, there are a variety of colors and products to choose from. Following is a guide to the different types of hair colors and how they work. Most hair colors come with explicit directions and you should follow them to the letter. We've included some additional tips on how to use specific products.

TEMPORARY RINSES

Rinses wake up dull hair color. They come in a wide variety of colors, from platinum to black to silver gray. A rinse is an excellent choice if you want to make gray or white hair look more vibrant. The color will wash out in the next shampoo.

SEMIPERMANENT AND PERMANENT HAIR COLORS

Semipermanent color coats the outside of the hair shaft and gradually washes out after about six to eight shampoos. It comes in shampoo-in and foam formulas. Using a semipermanent dye lets you experiment with color without making a commitment. It will brighten your hair and cover gray, but won't lighten it—so you won't have to worry about roots. It's also gentler on the hair than permanent color because it doesn't contain any peroxide. If you've never colored your hair before, you might want to start with a semipermanent color. The tone, however, tends to look a little flat. In addition, over a period of time, semipermanent color may collect on the ends of the hair. For this reason, it's good for layered hair. There won't be any buildup because you keep cutting off the ends of the hair.

Permanent hair color is the most natural looking and longest lasting. It contains peroxide, which can lighten or darken the hair to a greater degree than any other type of hair coloring. It doesn't wash out, but must grow out from the roots. When coloring your hair at home, you should use a single-process dye. This means that you apply the color in one step, usually by shampooing it in or applying a creamy formula. Avoid double-process hair colors, which are used to make the hair blond. Double processing involves prelightening the hair, then coloring with a toner. The two-step process is harsh and can damage the hair over time. If you have dark brown hair and would like to be blond, go to a professional colorist. At a good salon, the hair is made blond without double processing. It's lightened to a certain degree, then highlighted to avoid excessive damage.

CHOOSING THE RIGHT SHADE

A good general rule of thumb when selecting a hair color is to be brighter or a little lighter as you get older. For the most natural effect, you'll want to lift the color of your hair, without changing it drastically. When using a rinse or a semipermanent color, select a shade that's the same color or a shade lighter than your own hair. Choose permanent hair color that's one or two shades lighter than your hair. Remember that the lighter you go, the more of a maintenance program you'll be on. You will have to continue coloring your hair to cover dark roots.

If you have blond hair, avoid ash shades which can produce a greenish cast. Stick to wheat, platinum, golden or rosy tones, instead. On the other hand, when lightening medium to dark brown hair, red highlights may come out and the color may look brassy. If you don't want red highlights, choose an ash shade that's the same color as your hair, medium ash brown, for instance. If you want red highlights, choose auburn, cedar or wine shades. On dark to black hair, you can also pick a color in the red family just to make your hair shiny.

HIGHLIGHTING AND HAIR PAINTING

These techniques allow you to add brilliant highlights to your hair without making a drastic change. If you're just starting to go gray, they're a better alternative than dyeing all of your hair. Highlighting one-length hair is also healthier than dyeing it. The lightening agent used in these products is bleach. It strips the hair of color, but doesn't deposit any. When used properly, it can make your hair look sun-kissed. Another advantage: highlights require very little maintenance. You'll have to redo them only two or three times a year. And they look natural when growing out because there's no telltale root line.

FROSTING

Frosting produces a dramatic salt-and-pepper effect. Subtle highlights are more flattering, but if you like the look of frosting, go ahead and try it. Bleach is applied to selected strands of hair to make them a very light shade of blond. You'll get best results if you frost blond to light brown hair. On darker hair, blond highlights will create too much of a contrast.

GET YOUR HAIR GLOWING

Highlighting, hair painting and frosting kits come with everything you need to do the job yourself. Hair painting is done with a brush, but highlighting and frosting kits usually come with a cap. Very tiny strands of hair are pulled through the cap following a pattern designated in the kit's directions. To get the best results, concentrate on bleaching strands of hair framing the face and on top of the head where the sun would naturally hit. Touch the top layer of hair only and check frequently to see how the color is developing. Simply wipe the bleach off a strand of hair with a damp paper towel and examine it in sunlight to check the shade.

For very subtle highlights, leave the bleach on for only a short length of time. And never leave it on any longer than is recommended on the package. The next time you highlight or frost your hair, avoid rebleaching the same strands of hair. You could damage your hair or overlighten it. Instead, coat the already bleached strands with a thick conditioner and color new strands of hair.

HAIR LIGHTENERS

These products usually spray on and are used to bring out golden highlights, just as the sun would. Hair lighteners will brighten hair that's blond to light brown. But medium brown to black hair may turn a brassy shade of red. If you just want a slight color lift on light hair, apply a lightener for the minimum time recommended on the package. And be aware that your hair will get progressively lighter every time you apply it.

HENNA

Henna is a vegetable dye that has been used throughout history as a colorant. The ancient Egyptians used it to condition their hair. And the custom in the Middle East in olden times was to dye the palms of the hands and the soles of the feet with henna.

Henna coats the outside of the hair shaft and can result in a distinctive color change if you leave it on long enough. It won't wash out; you have to let it grow out. It comes in a variety of colors: blond, red, brown and black. Neutral henna, which is colorless, can be used to give body and luster to any shade of hair.

Colored hennas work best on medium brown to black hair. They'll bring out red highlights. Avoid dark colors of henna, which can look harsh. Stick to red shades. On medium brown hair, for instance, try strawberry blond henna. On dark brown hair, use an auburn shade. Aubergine will add a rich, deep glow to black hair. Never use colored henna on blond, light brown or gray hair—it will turn it bright red. If you just have a few gray hairs, however, henna will cover them up and create a tortoise-shell effect.

Look for pure natural henna. Some hennas contain metallic dyes that can cause an unpredictable color change. It can be hard to tell from the package whether or not henna is pure. Two brands you might try are Avigal and Hennalucent.

HENNA HOW-TOS

The directions that come with some hennas can be sketchy, so we've included explicit instructions on how to use it. Here are the steps to follow to get professional results. You'll need *a pair of rubber gloves* because henna can stain the skin, *a small hair-coloring brush* from a beauty supply store, *a wide-tooth plastic comb, a plastic cape* to catch spatters because henna can be runny, and *a glass or ceramic bowl* to mix henna. Never use a metal bowl or comb as both can have a bad reaction with henna.

Before applying henna, as an extra precaution, you should do a strand test to make sure you like the color. To do, mix a little henna with hot water until pasty. Apply it to a lock of hair in a spot that's not highly visible—behind the ear, for instance. Leave henna on for the full amount of time you would if you were doing a regular application (see step 7). Then wipe off the strand with a damp paper towel and check the results. If you're satisfied with the color, proceed according to the steps below.

1. Following package instructions, in a glass or ceramic bowl, mix henna to form a thick paste.
2. To apply it, you're going to follow the same procedure as for the blunt cut. Before you begin, cover the base of the neck and the shoulders with the cape to protect your skin. Starting in the back of the head, part hair from crown to nape. Comb down a diagonal wedge of hair 1 inch above the hairline. Dip the brush in the henna mixture. Beginning on the left side of the part, pick up a piece of hair, ½ inch thick, hold it out from the head at a 90-degree angle and paint it from roots to ends.

Work your way over to the left ear, picking up 1-inch-thick pieces of hair and painting them with henna. When you're done with the left side, comb hair sideways against the head to keep henna from running. Pick up 1-inch pieces of hair on the right, painting them from roots to ends until you've finished all the hair in that section.

3. Comb down another diagonal wedge 1 inch above the first. Divide it into smaller pieces and paint from top to bottom, always holding the hair out from the head. Work your way up to the crown, painting 1-inch-thick sections of hair from roots to ends, then combing them sideways on each side of the part to keep them off the neck.

4. Now go on and do one side of your hair. Comb down a horizontal section, 1 inch above the ear. Hold the hair straight out from the head or rest it on a gloved hand and paint from roots to ends. Slick the hair back against the side of the head after applying henna. Go up 1 inch and comb down another horizontal section of hair and paint the entire section.

5. Keep combing down horizontal sections of hair and painting them until you reach the part. Follow the same steps on the other side of the head.

6. Comb the hair away from the front hairline straight back and paint the roots of the hair.

7. Wrap up the hair in a towel or plastic bag and wait 40 minutes.

8. Shampoo the hair until the water runs clear. Henna is very grainy so you may have to wash it four or five times.

9. Condition the hair to remove any grains you might have missed.

CARE FOR COLOR-TREATED HAIR

Over time, coloring your hair with a dye, bleach or henna can make it more porous. If you don't care for your hair properly, it may become dryer and lose its elasticity. You must condition your hair regularly after you color it to keep it healthy. Use a good pH-balanced shampoo for your hair type. Because hair is more fragile, it may become tangled easily after shampooing. Use a light instant conditioner to unsnarl the hair and a deep conditioner twice a week if hair is brittle and damaged.

It's also important to protect color-treated hair from the sun. Sunlight can oxidize hair colorings. As a result, your hair may become too light or look brassy. In addition, bright sunlight can dry it out. An overdose of sun, in fact, can leave colored hair brittle and prone to breakage. When you're out in the sun, cover your head with a scarf, hat or cap in an open weave—it will protect your hair but let your scalp breathe. Although it may sound strange, it's also a good idea to protect your hair with a sunscreen. Use a cream-based sunscreen, as an alcohol-based one can be drying. Apply it lightly by running your fingers through your hair. Dab some sunscreen along your part line to prevent your scalp from getting burned, too. Chlorine and salt water can also be drying to the hair, so before you go swimming apply a coat of instant conditioner. Or wear a bathing cap to protect your hair. Afterward, rinse out chlorine or salt water and shampoo your hair. If you're not near a shower, take a misting bottle filled with water to the beach and spritz your hair.

QUESTIONS AND ANSWERS

Q. *How can I get rid of the dark fringe of hair over my upper lip?*

A. It's best to lighten the hair using a cream bleach available from a drugstore. Before applying it, do a patch test to make sure that your skin isn't sensitive to the bleaching solution. Apply a small amount in the crook of the elbow. Wait about 10 minutes, then rinse with cold water. If your skin doesn't become irritated within the next 24 hours, you can safely apply the bleach to your face, following the directions on the package label. Repeat the bleaching process every three weeks. If your skin is dark, avoid using bleach because it can lighten the skin as well. Try waxing instead, which is done at good salons. Another option is electrolysis, especially if facial hair is abundant. The procedure involves inserting a needle into the hair follicle, then sending an electric current through to destroy the roots. It should be done only by a licensed electrologist. Ask your doctor to recommend one.

Q. *My shoulder-length hair looks limp and stringy. It's oily at the roots and dry and split on the ends. How can I improve the condition of my hair without cutting it much shorter?*

A. Begin by trimming your hair to get rid of split ends. Wash it every day with a mild shampoo, making sure to cleanse the scalp thoroughly. Lightly suds the ends. Apply instant conditioner on the ends of the hair only. Brush daily with a natural-bristle brush to help distribute oils from the scalp down to the ends of the hair.

Q. *I got a perm about 10 days ago and now my scalp is flaky. I don't know if I have dandruff or if the chemicals in the perm caused this problem. What do you think?*

A. Your perm was probably overprocessed and left on too long.

As a result, your scalp has become dry and flaky. What your hair needs is moisture. Use a deep conditioner on your hair after every shampoo and leave it on for 5 to 10 minutes. Follow this conditioning program until your scalp returns to normal. Also use a shampoo made especially for dry or damaged hair.

Q. *My hair is fragile and fine and looks lifeless. I use a body-building conditioner and shampoo but my hair starts to wilt a few hours after I've washed it. How can I make it look thicker?*

A. A layered style that's no longer than the base of the neck can make your hair appear fuller. Also consider getting a body wave, which will give the hair more volume. Make sure to have your hair trimmed regularly to increase body and bounce.

Q. *I've been lightening my hair for several years and it's dull, dry and brittle. Is there any way to make it soft and shiny again?*

A. Your hair is overworked. Applying an intensive conditioner such as a protein pack or a hot oil treatment once a week will help restore your hair's resiliency and shine. Try switching to a non-peroxide hair color, which is gentler on the hair than a permanent dye. Keep blow-drying to a minimum. It can further dry out damaged hair. And make sure to handle your hair with care. Don't pull or tug at it while shampooing. To avoid breakage, comb and brush the hair carefully.

Q. *My hair is dry and flyaway. How can I make it more manageable?*

A. The best thing you can do for flyaway hair is to condition it. Use a cream rinse or a light conditioner after shampooing. Avoid heavy conditioners, which can overload your hair. Never use a brush with plastic bristles and a rubber base. It will add static electricity to your hair. Instead use a natural-bristle brush with a wooden base.

Q. *I recently had a baby and my hair has become much thinner. Every time I brush it, more falls out. I'm getting worried. Could this condition be permanent?*

A. Hair loss after pregnancy is quite common. The hormonal changes your body has experienced have caused more of your hair to go into a resting phase. Hair grows in cycles—long growing periods followed by short resting phases in which hair stops growing and falls out. Your hair will grow back in time. Meanwhile, stop brushing and comb your hair gently instead. You want to avoid putting any additional stress on your hair.

Q. *After several weeks of swimming without a bathing cap, my hair, a light shade of blond, developed a greenish tinge. What causes this and what can I do about it?*

A. Copper sulfate algaecides—chemicals added to disinfect swimming pools—cling to the hair shaft and cause discoloration on light-colored hair. To prevent the problem, use a special anti-chlorine shampoo and conditioner made for swimmers that will protect the hair and prevent any color change. Wearing a bathing cap when you go swimming will help, too. And make sure to shampoo your hair afterward to remove pool chemicals.

Q. *I have fine, naturally curly hair. During humid weather, it gets frizzy and hard to control. Why does this happen and how can I make my hair behave?*

A. When the humidity is high, your hair absorbs moisture from the air, which makes the hair shaft swell. As a result, your hair may stick out or look wiry. To fight frizzies, use a light conditioner after every shampoo to make the hair lie down smoothly. Then to keep it under control, apply mousse or gel before styling. If frizzies pop up during the middle of the day, here's a quick way to get rid of them: put a dime-sized dollop of mousse or gel into your hand and smooth down the outer layer of your hair with your palms.

Q. *I often get ingrown hairs as a result of shaving. What's the best way to prevent this problem?*

A. Shaving against the grain and shaving too closely are the two main causes of ingrown hairs. Men with coarse, curly hair are prone to this problem. The hair curves inward after shaving and becomes imbedded in the skin. Make sure to use a sharp blade when shaving and alway shave in the direction in which the hair grows. Using a new blade for each shave will ensure a smooth, clean shave. Another alternative is to stop shaving and grow a beard. If the skin becomes irritated from an ingrown hair, see a dermatologist.